BRITISH MEDICINE IN AN AGE OF REFORM

THE WELLCOME INSTITUTE SERIES IN THE HISTORY OF MEDICINE

Edited by W.F. Bynum and Roy Porter,

The Wellcome Institute

Medical Fringe and Medical Orthodoxy, 1750–1850
W.F. Bynum and Roy Porter
Florence Nightingale and the Nursing Legacy
Monica Baly
Social Hygiene in Twentieth Century Britain
Greta Jones
Problems and Methods in the History of Medicine
Roy Porter and Andrew Wear
Vivisection in Historical Perspective
Nicolaas A. Rupke
(Now available in paperback)
Abortion in England, 1919–1967
Barbara Brookes
The Hospital in History
Edited by Lindsay Granshaw and Roy Porter
(Now available in paperback)
Women as Mothers in Pre-Industrial England
Edited by Valerie Fildes
Birth Control in Germany, 1871–1933
James Woycke
The Charitable Imperative
Colin Jones
Medicine at the Courts of Europe, 1500–1837
Edited by Dr Vivian Nutton
Mad Tales from the Raj
Waltraud Ernst

BRITISH MEDICINE IN AN AGE OF REFORM

Edited by Roger French and Andrew Wear

ROUTLEDGE
London and New York

First published in 1991
by Routledge
11 New Fetter Lane, London EC4P 4EE

Simultaneously published in the USA and Canada
by Routledge
a division of Routledge, Chapman and Hall Inc.
29 West 35th Street, New York, NY 10001

Typeset by LaserScript, Mitcham, Surrey
Printed in Great Britain by Biddles Ltd, Guildford and King's Lynn

British Library Cataloguing in Publication Data

British medicine in an age of reform.
1. Great Britain. Medicine, history
I. French, Roger II. Wear, Andrew III. Series
610.941

Library of Congress Cataloging in Publication Data

British medicine in an age of reform/edited by Roger French and Andrew Wear.
p. cm. – (The Wellcome series in the history of medicine)
Based on a conference held Sept. 1987 in London and sponsored by the Royal Institution's Centre for the History of Science and Technology.
Includes bibliographical references and index.
1. Medicine – Great Britain – History – 18th century – Congresses.
2. Medicine – Great Britain – History – 19th century – Congresses.
I. French, R.K. (Roger Kenneth) II. Wear, A. (Andrew), 1946–
III Royal Institution Centre for the History of Science and Technology. IV. Series.
[DNLM: 1. History of Medicine, 18th Century – Great Britain – congresses. 2. History of Medicine, 19th Century – Great Britain – congresses. WZ 70 FA1 B85 1987]
R487.B75 1991
610'.941'09033 – dc20
DNLM/DLC
90-9163
CIP

ISBN 0–415–05622–5

Contents

Tables and figures

Tables

Figures

Editors and contributors

Editors

Roger French is Director of the Wellcome Unit for the History of Medicine, University of Cambridge.

Andrew Wear is Lecturer at the Wellcome Institute for the History of Medicine, London.

Contributors

Logie Barrow is Professor of British Social History in the department of Sprach- und Kulturwissenschaften, University of Bremen, Germany.

Catherine Crawford is a Wellcome Research Lecturer in the History department, University of Essex.

Mary Fissell is Research Associate at the Wellcome Unit for the History of Medicine, University of Manchester.

Elizabeth Haigh is Professor of History at Saint Mary's University, Halifax, Canada.

Stephen Jacyna is Research Officer at the Wellcome Unit for the History of Medicine, University of Manchester.

Susan Lawrence is in the department of History, University of Iowa, Iowa City, Iowa.

Roy Porter is Senior Lecturer at the Wellcome Institute for the History of Medicine, London.

Ruth Richardson is at the Institute of Historical Research, University of London.

John Harley Warner is Associate Professor of the History of Medicine, Yale University, New Haven, Connecticut.

Perry Williams is in the Wellcome Unit for the History of Medicine, University of Cambridge.

Acknowledgements

We are grateful to the Royal Institution's Centre for the History of Science and Technology, which was host to the conference that gave rise to this book. We are also grateful for financial support from the Wellcome Trust.

Introduction

British medicine changed radically in the seventy years or so that preceded the middle of the nineteenth century. This was the Age of Reform, in medicine as in politics. By the end of the period, the shape of medicine as a profession was recognizably modern. The content, the teaching, and the practice of medicine also changed extensively, although they did not become so 'modern' until the adoption of the Germ Theory in the later nineteenth century.

The chapters of this book bring into prominence a number of narratives that are aspects of this change. Roy Porter's chapter sets the scene for change and explores an early call for reform, that of Thomas Beddoes. Beddoes was above all an individual – radical, eccentric, and seeking, unlike his colleagues, to improve the doctor–patient relationship by reforming the patient. Lone voices rarely effect change, and another narrative of this book is that of external change – institutional change imposed from without – such as the Apothecaries' Act, the Anatomy Act, and finally the Medical Act at the very end of our period. Third, there was pressure for reform from within the profession, directed not only against the old medical corporations, but towards a new style of teaching. Thus, the content of medical knowledge changed: it became 'scientific'. While many of the voices in favour of change were those of individuals, where change of whatever kind took place it was within groups of people, in hospitals, in the universities, in the medical corporations, and in the private schools. The scale of such change was achieved only by the interested parties securing parliamentary help. Parliament was concerned with reform on a much wider scale, and medical reform was part of a wider movement. The *laissez-faire* approach to government that characterized Britain in the eighteenth century was increasingly challenged in the nineteenth century by a more centralized and interventionist view of government. In medicine there was an analogous switch from the largely unregulated open market-place of the eighteenth century to increasingly regulated medical education and practice.

Let us try to sketch the broad lines of the changes that are dealt with in these chapters. With the hindsight of the 1858 Medical Act, which established and regulated the modern-sounding general practitioner as the dominant type of medical man (although the general practitioners of the time were disappointed with the Act), the medicine of the late eighteenth century appeared fragmented. The ancient English universities had privileges in licensing their graduates that dated from the thirteenth and fourteenth centuries, but gave very little instruction. In Scotland, Edinburgh continued to teach and license extensively, while Aberdeen licensed for a fee and on scant evidence of training. The private anatomy schools flourished, but their courses were not always recognized. The old medical corporations had regulatory powers within their branches of the profession that had resulted from guild or college negotiating from the crown monopoly which was limited and in the eighteenth century often ignored. Medical theory, after the breakdown of the Boerhaavian consensus by mid-century, was fragmented between the different systems of the nosologists, the echoes of the mid-century dispute between animists and mechanists, and more recent reductionist theories of bodily action. The well-read, well-heeled patient of the physician may well have played a part in the decision about his disease and its treatment. Medicine was also fragmented between the towns, where alone the physician could find a sufficient density of fee-paying patients to support himself in style, and the country, where the indigence of rural folk had long rendered meaningless the distinctions between the branches of the profession and the claims of the old corporations to control it.

By the 1780s Britain was imperial and increasingly industrial. Urbanization and increasing wealth were economic changes that had far-reaching social and ultimately medical effects. Thomas Beddoes (in Roy Porter's chapter) saw the 'civilization' of the growing towns itself as a source of sickness. But Britain was an island in a maritime sense only, not economically and politically. The French Revolution seemed to many to be the realization of a Enlightenment dream of the liberation of man. To others, its example seemed dangerously subversive of the established order. When revolutionary France began to threaten Britain's imperial connections there was cause for even greater concern at home. Repression might cause revolution; reform might defuse it.

For reasons of equality and of military effectiveness the distinction between physician and surgeon was abolished in France and the profession was placed under more centralized control than that in Britain. Medical teaching and practice, centred in large hospitals, came to have a number of characteristics absent from English medicine. Large numbers of patients were available in the same place. Physical elicitation of signs became characteristic of the examination of the patient. Systematic post-mortem dissection of the patient was used to relate these signs to the diseased state of the body. Morbid – pathological – anatomy became the centrepin of medical theory and research.

In contrast, British medicine retained many of its eighteenth-century characteristics. The hospitals were comparatively small and the doctor could not make wide-ranging comparisons. The physician, calling on his well-to-do client at home, still negotiated with him about his disease and its treatment. In this case as well as lower down the profession, the medical man based his treatment on what the patient told him about his illness, rather than on signs he could make the patient's body give. Post-mortem dissection was not linked to such signs. Pathology remained morbid physiology rather than becoming morbid anatomy.

British medicine changed partly in response to the new French medicine. As Stephen Jacyna points out, this was not a passive reception, but a selective interpretation based on the individual's extant knowledge, perceptions, and requirements. After the Napoleonic wars the individuals going to France for its medicine became a flood, and the travelling Scots described by Jacyna took home a perception of French medicine that was partly shaped by their own Scottish concerns with the organization of hospitals and with the need to improve surgical education. The letters of the two Scots studied by Jacyna show how the French model of pathological anatomy could be viewed as part of clinical medicine or as a discipline in its own right.

British medicine changed for domestic reasons too. Reform that would avert revolution or create a more just society (depending on whence it was viewed) had to be a reform of society's institutions, including the medical. Susan Lawrence gives an account of the Apothecaries' Act, the first initiative (1815) through Parliament towards control of the medical profession. The Apothecaries' power to define what a medical course was gave some structure to the characteristic London situation of competing private medical courses and teaching within the hospitals. Lawrence shows how the Apothecaries were initially flexible when it came to the courses and medical experience required of the candidate for a licence. Increasingly, however, they closed the open market in education. They decided which courses were acceptable for the licence and assigned greater importance to hospital than to dispensaries by requiring longer attendance in the latter. London was gradually being pushed in the direction of the new French regulated medicine, with its emphasis on hospital teaching, which encouraged the study of morbid anatomy.

Another domestic change in British medicine was the Anatomy Act of 1832, described in this volume by Ruth Richardson. Concerned more with controlling the supply of dissection material to the anatomy schools than with any French notion of morbid anatomy, it was handled (in close proximity to the Reform Bill) by Parliament in a reforming way. The Anatomy Inspectorate was the first of many Benthamite, centrally conceived bodies that began to govern different aspects of the nation's commercial and professional life. Reforming actions were of their nature concerned with the problems of one or more disadvantaged groups. In this case, the anatomists lacked cadavers (and the dead were robbed of their graves and the innocent murdered to provide material for dissection). The disadvantaged poor, whose bodies were not claimed by close relations, were to supplement executed criminals as a source of cadavers for dissection. As in France, but in a rather different way, the poor became the objects of research in pathological anatomy. In a wider sense, the Act came to serve the political purpose of deterring people from entering the workhouse by making it an even more dreaded institution.

Calls for reform came from below, or from the champions of the underprivileged, as well as from the Benthamite social engineers. Within medicine the underprivileged were the young, or those without hope of entering the old corporations and practising at the highest level. Their champion was Wakley and his weapon the *Lancet*. Also outside established medicine were those practising a kind of medicine not approved of by the universities, professional colleges, and reformers of 'regular' medicine. Their relationship to reform is discussed by Logie Barrow. This chapter reminds us that alternative medicine (in contrast to eighteenth century empiricism based on the individual practitioner), developed in the nineteenth century, with its own sects and organizations analogous to those of regular medicine, represented a strong force opposing the newly emerging form of scientific medicine.

One major change that overcame medicine in this period has not yet been discussed. It became scientific. Now, rational medicine, the medicine of the learned physician, had been based, since the Middle Ages, on natural philosophy. It was indeed by means of natural philosophy that the medieval physician both justified the inclusion of his subject within the university and impressed his wealthy and educated patients. It was on the changing natural philosophies of the eighteenth century that medicine – also changing – was still based, whether Galenic, chemical, mechanical, animistic, or Brunonian. But natural philosophy was not science. It was, to be sure, a *scientia*, like mathematics, theology, or geography, but it did not have the characteristics of science as we think of it. Its foundations and purpose were different, and for Boyle and Newton, as for the philosophers and deists of the eighteenth century, it was about the actions of God in a created world. But Enlightenment thought and revolution were increasingly about humanity, and historians have recognized a 'de-Christianization' of philosophy in the later eighteenth century. (Although this term is not used by our colleague Andrew Cunningham, we should like to thank him for many useful discussions on what he has called, in a recent number of *Studies in History and Philosophy of Science*, 'the invention of science'.)

It is only in the early nineteenth century that people use the term 'science' to stand on its own and not to indicate knowledge, *scientia*, of a specialized kind. And it is only at this time, too, that there comes into existence a class of people who were occupied principally in pursuit of 'science', professional 'scientists'. Of course it is tempting, from the viewpoint of the scientific medicine of the late nineteenth century, which was suddenly so effective in controlling some infectious diseases, to see that the seeds of that effectiveness were laid early in the century, when medicine became scientific. However, as the following chapters show, 'science' was a term coined partly in the rhetoric of reform. It meant, moreover, very different things to different people.

When Babbage in 1830 urged reform by arguing that science in England had decayed, he was, as John Harley Warner shows, using an argument that had about a ten-year history and a word, 'science', that was not much older. The argument and the word were used by the general practitioners. They did not have the social breeding of the physicians or access to their genteel and wealthy patients. They accordingly argued for the superiority of their own kind of medicine by calling it 'scientific' and saw it as a means of substituting meritocracy for social rank. What they meant was the new French medicine they had seen in their travels to Paris: physical elicitation of signs, large hospitals, systematic post-mortem examination, and morbid anatomy. Though the British were confident that their practical therapeutics were superior to those of the French, whom they accused of doing nothing for their patients, they believed that the French were far superior in their scientific diagnosis. While the gentlemanly doctor still listened to and acted upon the narrative of his disease by the patient, the effect of French practice, as Mary Fissell shows even for provincial Bristol, was that the patient's narrative disappeared. Early in the eighteenth century the patient's and the doctor's narrative of illness had a certain symmetry, aspects of one being included in the other. Towards the end of the century doctors' accounts of illness were increasingly divorced from lay language, and, for example, Latin rapidly replaced English. The patient in a voluntary hospital did not pay the doctor and was one of a large number. His or her social standing and education were inferior to those of the doctor. For all these reasons, the doctor was less disposed to put reliance on what the patient said; moreover, he now had his own physical means of procuring signs from the patient's body, signs that in relating to the scientificness of medicine were thought superior to the patient's unlearned story of his own disease. (That orthodox and scientific doctors seemed to ignore their patients, as Logie Barrow points out, gave the unorthodox an advantage in emphasizing personal contact.)

Thus, 'science' in medicine was partly what English practitioners of the middling sort felt that they could take from a French example to help them reform medicine, that is, to encroach on the ground of the learned and gentlemanly physicians. The utility of French medicine for similar purposes was seen by Americans in Paris, and they too took back home French 'science'. But it was different from the science talked about by English general practitioners, for the Americans (because of the nature of other parts of the domestic profession) found it scientific to denounce rationalism and emphasize sensual empiricism.

So, in Britain, science was largely associated with medicine (certainly the medical men composed the biggest category of scientific people), it was meritocratic and democratic, it implied state support for training, and it claimed superiority on the basis of French methods of investigation. A not dissimilar story is told by Elizabeth Haigh. Animal chemistry was science, partly because it was of interest to the medical man. Chemistry was of natural interest to the apothecary, the new general practitioner of the earlier part of the century. The study of chemistry itself was as scientific as medicine in being a means whereby the meritocratic lower-middle-class practitioner could raise his status in relation to the gentlemanly physician.

The growth of forensic medicine in England in the first half of the nineteenth century was clearly allied to medical reform and to medical science. Wakley wrote that the quality of the medical evidence given in a country's law courts was the best indicator of the state of its medical science. Catherine Crawford shows how the ideals of a new gentlemanly, utilitarian and scientific medicine were appealed to by journal editors and others, and how in reality these ideals often failed to materialize. The medical community was acutely embarrassed by the public disagreements of medical experts in the courts, since scientific forensic medicine formed part of the reformers' campaign of eliminating the uncertainty of unreformed medicine: an uncertainty which, it was agreed, had proved fertile ground for the empiric and charlatan.

Reform in medicine also took place in nursing and this too is part of the story of how medicine became modern. Perry Williams poses the novel question of why nurses began to be seen as needing reform, when, in the eighteenth century and earlier, the position of nurses as lowly servants in houses or institutions was taken for granted. Hospital governors and then religiously motivated reformers pressed for change. The latter intended that British nurses should be Protestant versions of the Catholic orders of nuns, an intention that was an expression of religious charity from the enthusiastic religion of eighteenth-century dissenters to the Victorian religious revival. In the process of implementing this intention a new reformed nurse was created, who was to be guided by the middle-class ideals of femininity rather than by any model of science derived from France. Without a male education, she could be no threat to the other parts of the medical profession. Without a knowledge of science, based on a French rationality that could easily lead to scepticism, the 'sisters' of the Protestant order were secure in their calling. To accompany the new nurse there was created the image of the unreformed past, epitomized by Dickens's Sarah Gamp.

Our period represents a major watershed in British medicine. The contributions to this book should help to throw light on the nature and the dynamics of the changes that were involved.

1

Reforming the patient in the age of reform: Thomas Beddoes and medical practice

Roy Porter

In the age of reform, one of the institutions thought ripest for reformation was medicine. Endless meetings were addressed and pamphlets published promoting that cause, and the ensuing modernization of medicine has generally been seen as a self-evidently good thing.[1] After all, was not the old order vitiated by closed, oligarchic corporations, the decay of medical education, whether at Oxbridge or in the antiquated apprenticeship system for training common practitioners, by a paucity of qualified doctors, and certainly by a lack of skill – while all the time the toadstool millionaires were left to multiply unchecked? By contrast, the new order the reformers eventually succeeded in building was graced by more meritocratic colleges, the emergence of the family doctor, the parliamentary enforcement of minimum entry requirements, the marginalization of the unqualified, the establishment of the Medical Register and the General Medical Council, and the brisk new professionalism of the British Medical Association, the *British Medical Journal*, and the *Lancet*: improvement all round.

Just how far – or, better, perhaps, how *little* – today's historians can accept this traditional tableau of reform triumphant is a crucial question for this book as a whole – one which will not, however, be further explored here.[2] My aim, rather, is to examine a particular neglected facet of the reformist agenda.

Thanks to the researches of Sidney Holloway, Ivan Waddington, Irvine Loudon, and others, we are now better informed about the aims and claims of ordinary provincial practitioners in the decades from the 1790s, and about the activities of their central spokesmen, such as Thomas Wakley, founder of the *Lancet*.[3] They wanted to change medicine from above and below. At its head, the medical colleges formed one target: their portals must be opened or their teeth must be drawn. At its foot, cowboy practice had to be ended, quackery outlawed, or, at least, empirics regularized. In this recent historiography of medical modernization, which sheds new light upon the aspirations and interests of the practitioners themselves, one reformist drive has, however, remained ignored: the desire to reform the patient.

Medical historians long neglected the dynamics of bedside practice. Then, in the 1970s, our understanding of the history of patient/doctor relations was significantly advanced by the sociologist Nicholas Jewson, who contended for the influential role of the (wealthy) patient in pre-1800 clinical medicine.[4] Drawing upon Jewson's pioneer, if rather abstract, articles, empirical investigations have subsequently been laying bare the micro-politics of common-or-garden practice, seen 'from below' or 'from the patient's point of view'. We now have a richer grasp of a traditional, client-orientated system, in which attention was granted to the sick person's own 'history', diagnostic hunches, and even therapeutic preferences.[5] These were the tacit norms – professional, cognitive, and commercial – within which practitioners typically had to operate, like it or not. But what did doctors think about such terms of service? How did they regard their clients? And how, and how far, did they want clinical relations to change?

Obviously, those campaigning to curb quacks and correct the colleges pledged heartfelt concern for the welfare of the sick as their motive. But, aside from noting such ideological anodynes, doctors' attitudes towards patients have been little studied. Or, more precisely, a certain rather general viewpoint has recently been gaining ground. Teasing out the implications of Jewson's hypothesis of the 'disappearance of the sick man from medical cosmology', and extending Foucault's insights about the enhanced cognitive authority of hospital medicine from around 1800,[6] it is now often suggested that the sick person, like the Cheshire cat, faded from the doctor's vision. The ailing human being, with his 'complaints', was replaced by a new *Gestalt*, that of a body suffering from various lesions, whose signs the practitioner would investigate, increasingly as the century wore on, using diagnostic technology, and thus setting less store by the patient's own story. Mary Fissell's contribution to this volume, 'The disappearance of the patient's narrative and the invention of hospital medicine', offers a convincing demonstration of this very process at work, in context of the 'clinic'.[7]

There is a truth in this, yet it is far from the whole story, and it would be a shame if the Jewson-Foucault interpretation became an excuse for renewed scholarly indifference to the sick person, or rather to the clinical duo. The sympathies and loyalties of reforming doctors in respect of their patients were often complex. If they frequently resented them as ignoramuses or tiresome busybodies, they could also feel common cause with common people in combating oppression, privilege, and corruption. The modern doctor, the reforming doctor, did not solely want his patients to shut up, lie back, and submit to the medical gaze. So what *did* practitioners think of their patients, actual and idealized, past, present, and future? In this chapter I shall focus upon the views of one single physician, Thomas Beddoes.

Thomas Beddoes

Beddoes was an outspoken, no-nonsense maverick, a radical facing the future with more than a tinge of nostalgia for the plain and simple past. His career was unconventional and somewhat chequered. Born in 1760, this Shropshire lad took his BA at Oxford and then pursued medicine at Edinburgh, before becoming a pioneer of chemistry teaching at his *alma mater.* Vilified for his outspoken pro-French Revolution and anti-Pitt politics, Beddoes quit Oxford, removing to practise in the Bristol suburb of Clifton, where he opened his Pneumatic Institute in 1799. Initially established to further scientific therapeutics, the Institute dwindled into a more general receptacle for the 'sick and drooping poor'. Beddoes meantime earned his living by treating a fashionable clientele. He thus acquired extensive face-to-face experience with a broad band of sufferers.[8]

For a decade and a half from the early 1790s, Beddoes produced a stream of works addressed to reforming medicine.[9] Unlike many of his contemporaries, he was not primarily concerned with reorganizing the superstructure of the profession and its statutory basis. He principally wanted to improve the politics of health at the contact point of doctor–patient relations and, more broadly, to set health care and medical practice on more fruitful footings.

Beddoes's directives towards the poor, such as *The History of Isaac Jenkins, and of the Sickness of Sarah his Wife, and Their Three Children* (1792), are the staple admonitory pabulum of the times. Be thrifty, be frugal, be industrious, be regular, be clean, be hardy, be continent, be temperate, and, above all else, be sober. Beddoes instructed the labouring classes in a prose which narrowly escapes Hannah More's egregiously patronizing incantations. Beddoes's priority was to teach the indigent habits which would strengthen their health and so minimize the need for doctoring. I shall not explore these writings further here.[10]

By contrast, Beddoes wrote with zest, originality, and umbrage about medicine among the polite and propertied in a series of wordy works, above all *Hygeia*,[11] first published in eleven monthly instalments from 1802 to 1803 and running to some 1500 pages, and the *Manual of Health* (1807),[12] a mere five hundred pages. Both were targeted at the 'middle and more opulent classes',[13] for they alone, Beddoes observed, had the 'necessary degree of intelligence'.[14] His professed aim in these works and elsewhere was to expose defects in the daily practice of doctoring – the covetousness of practitioners,[15] the cozenings of quacks,[16] and, above all, the follies of the affluent classes themselves, in health and in sickness – in the hope that readers, suitably chastened, would mend their ways.

Civilization and its sicknesses

Improvement was in the air.[17] The bracing breezes of freedom, inquiry, and criticism (so ran a familiar Enlightenment rhetoric) were fanning the advancement of useful and practical knowledge. Medicine itself, Beddoes believed, had been transformed by the Scientific Revolution. He personally played some part in the 'chemical revolution', and at one exhilarating stage in his career proffered positively millennial hopes of curing all manner of fatal diseases through the use of laboratory-produced gases, announcing 'a great revolution in this art is at hand'. Did Beddoes then think that the progress of enlightenment and science were bearing fruit in tangible health improvements, affording still more rosy prospects for the future? Far from it.[18]

Beddoes's writings for the intelligent layman present a uniformly bleak picture of sufferings and setbacks. Such traditional illnesses as scarlatina and other fevers continued unabated, endangering even the wealthy. Other fatal diseases were newly rampant, above all, tuberculosis. And a host of chronic conditions, perhaps not lethal but disabling none the less, were also growing worse: gout, nervous maladies, scrofula, mental derangement, hysteria, hypochondria, indigestive disorders, and general debility. Beddoes had no doubts about where to point the blame: 'our chronic maladies are of our creating'.[19]

Nor was there cause for complacency on the medical front. Few successful cures had been discovered: Beddoes's own hopes for oxygen as a panacea were soon to be dashed. Worse, Beddoes believed that the medical profession itself had become hopelessly corrupted by the temptations of trade and the lure of lucre, and that, partly as a result, quackery was raging out of control.[20] Surveying the 'sick trade', he saw rampant everywhere the 'grossness of medical impostures', regular and irregular alike, hoodwinking even 'people who have enjoyed the most liberal education', in their fight to gain 'the privilege of lucrative homicide'.[21]

So why was progress proving pathological? Beddoes was neither a reactionary nor a Rousseauvian. He did not believe in original sin or that the civilizing process necessarily spelt a fall from some pristine natural state of health, happiness, or holiness. Hence, for a progressive of his kidney, the signs of deterioration in health, and, perhaps, also in medicine, required explanation and rectification. The heart of the matter, Beddoes believed, lay in the massive transformations effected by commerce during the Georgian era, in creating a 'society in its complicated state'.[22]

Fundamental was the growth of affluence. 'In the social arrangements which have gradually formed themselves in Europe', he observed, 'WEALTH, the most general object of power, becomes the most general object of desire.'[23] The multiplication of wealth was creating a restless, emulative, achiever society, new conveniences and luxuries in domestic and urban life-styles, greater freedom in living ('in no country is there so large a proportion of inhabitants with such liberty of choice, as in Great Britain'),[24] super-sophisticated manners, and a broadening of personal, intellectual, and literary horizons – those currents we may call the Enlightenment.[25] Such otherwise desirable developments, Beddoes believed, were threatening to sap well-being itself. But he was also anxious to show how, perhaps more alarmingly, they were also warping attitudes towards health, hamstringing abilities to cope with sickness, and sabotaging therapeutic relations between patients and practitioners.

Britain, Beddoes reflected in 1802, took pride in its freedom, its international commercial and military power, its riches. Yet, 'Is all this solid benefit or empty boast?' He doubted whether such developments produced solid and lasting benefit. 'What revenue of health and comfort has our vast dominion over art and nature yielded? . . . One may account the pride of power as the same thing, in effect, to the body politic, with intense, enervating pleasure to the body natural. Has Britain wasted her vigour in the debauches of glory?' – indeed, was Britain due to suffer, as widely prophesied, an imminent 'millennium of misery'?[26]

The problem lay in the ascendancy of commercial commodity capitalism. In numerous works, Beddoes revealed how the manufacturing system destroyed the health of workers, cooped up in cramped, polluted workshops, exposed to noxious fumes and dust, and condemned to sedentariness. 'The encouragement of manufactures', he remarked in *Hygeia*, 'is the creation of a miserable and sickly population.'[27] But commerce was hardly less unhealthy for the employing classes, all too often rendered sickly by 'early confinement in compting-houses' in dark-roomed towns which 'abridged health'.[28] Beddoes particularly deprecated the growing habit among the business classes of 'sacrific[ing] their offspring to Moloch', by putting out their sons as merchants' clerks at far too tender an age: their fate? – to end up with ruined stomachs as hypochondriacs.[29]

The bilious, however, got off lightly. For financial speculation was all too liable to drive its votaries to utter distraction.[30] 'Go for instance to the scenes of trade at London or at Bristol', Beddoes urged the sceptical:

> Among the faces that appear at high 'Change, mark those that bespeak the cares attendant upon wealth already accumulated; and those others, where an added air of wildness characterises the speculator, too much in haste to wait for the reward of regular industry, and burning to get rich by the lucky hit. Some of these men will grow mad enough to be watched at home or sent to a lunatic asylum,

where they will be haunted by the fear of coming upon the parish.[31]

But greed for gold destroyed the health not only of businessmen. The opportunity society[32] created unease, anxiety, and dissatisfaction for everyone consumed by getting and spending. Money was itself a devil. 'The universal facility of credit in this country', Beddoes alleged, was often disastrous for health, especially perhaps for 'those students who are in haste to ruin their constitution'.[33] Easy credit today, deep indebtedness tomorrow, sometimes with fatal consequences.[34] *'All the world is melancholy, because all the world is in debt'* – this commonplace 'observation', Beddoes reflected, 'certainly, will not account for the whole of the melancholy among us. . . . But it will account for a great many of those unwelcome visitations, against which no gaiety of apparel is able to protect many a snowy bosom.'[35]

Primitive societies might suffer worse from acute disorders, but urban affluence, and its 'over-fondness for the *good things* of life', proved the seedbed for terrible new chronic malaises;[36] perhaps grief was in order 'as much for the fate of those who consume as of those who manufacture various articles of luxury'.[37] Modern man had generated monstrous desires and wants, above all 'a taste for more refined luxuries'; with these he could not cope, for 'the appetite is found too strong for the mind, and for the body too'.[38]

Beddoes was thus distressed by the physical evils of acquisitiveness and the consequent diseases of civilization. 'The English', he noted, 'are more remarkable than any other nation on the globe for the accumulation of *comforts*, and indeed unhappily we pique ourselves upon the distinction.'[39] Why 'unhappily'? Though dismissing the draconian solution – that the reader should 'discard his or her comforts all at once' – it was his intention, Beddoes insisted, to 'open a course of reflexion', thanks to which they might 'satisfy themselves that the reliance they place on externals is vain'. Readers should ponder the seeming paradox that 'those who have most comforts about them, are commonly the most comfortless of all mortals',[40] for 'those who want nothing else very commonly want health'.[41]

Numerous facets of an economy blessed, or cursed, with surplus wealth, and addicted to the pleasures of property and the comforts of 'passive enjoyments',[42] proved especially damaging to health, both physical and mental. Like many an earlier medical moralist, steeped in the age-old rhetoric of civic humanism, Beddoes was the sworn foe to luxury.[43] But, unlike George Cheyne a couple of generations earlier, Beddoes did not take as his target gross gluttony and drunkenness.[44] For that gargantuan personal consumption condemned by Cheyne, who himself weighed in at 32 stone, had itself seemingly undergone its own civilizing process, becoming more refined – now one ate 'sauces as kill hunger by inches'[45] – but thereby all the more insidious, because greed had camouflaged itself in the decorous idiom of politeness.

Nowadays the buzz of background chat at dinners ran rather as follows: '" – do let me send you some more of this mock turtle" – "another paté" – "Sir, some of the trifle", "a few slices of cucumber" – "I SHALL INSIST upon your trying this nice melon".' Better by far to drop these genteel pretences, and to talk straight about the health risks involved. Translate into bluff medical lingo: '"shall I send you a fit of the cholic" – "do let me help you to a little bilious vomiting and purging" – "Ma'am, you cannot refuse a touch of inflammation in the bowels – It may come to a tight race between your intestines and your physician. But I hope it will stop before it gets quite to the undertaker and the sexton".'[46]

Luxury – or even a life devoted to ease – was a false idol: 'every half hour, spent out of the carpeted, stuccoed, and stoved sitting room, will contribute towards the redemption of the constitution from oppressive languor and sickliness.'[47] Worse, it was attended by, and contributory to, other evils. For one thing, there was the vertiginous hurry of modern life, growing ever faster, more hectic, and confused. '*Did you see the papers today? Have you read the new play – the new poem – the new pamphlet – the last novel?*' was all that was heard these days. 'You cannot creditably frequent intelligent company, without being prepared to answer these questions, and the progeny that springs from them.' The consequence? 'You must needs hang your heavy head, and roll your bloodshot eyes over thousands of pages weekly. Of their contents at the week's end, you will know about as much as of a district, through which you have been whirled night and day in the mail-coach.' Headachy exhaustion was the toll of all this 'quick desultory reading': 'What wonder then that we should hear complaints against the age as wanting energy of feeling and compass of mind?'[48]

Fast living and the itch for novelty – the two phrases on every pair of polite lips were *'as soon as possible'* and *'as fast as possible!'*[49] – reinforced competitive, emulative life-styles and the urge to live in the eyes of the world, seeing and being seen. 'An universal interest must be taken in the condition of those about us, not less lively than the desire we see so prevalent of dazzling strangers by the splendour of an equipage or by the lights of the understanding.' We crave admiration, wanting to have 'every thing about us – cloaths, tables, chairs, pictures, statues – all exquisite in their kind'; the only thing neglected in all this sumptuous parade is our health, and that of our children. We ought to be 'shocked at seeing, under the same roof, perfect representations of the human figure' – that is, statues and paintings – 'in contrast with the most wretched realities. . . . Parents, in short, must find and seek honour in the healthiness of their children.'[50]

The demon here was, of course, fashion, that 'fawning, treacherous divinity'.[51] This 'despotism of fancy' was the greatest, and most degenerate, despotism of all: 'what elicits . . . sparks of emulation from the eyes, and induces agitations that equally disturb the rest, of thousands of striplings and of damsels, panting for celebrity in Britain? – why, may be, a nosegay of artificial plumes, or a well stiffened collar.'[52] Indeed, in the carnage of civilization, he noted, presumably glancing sidelong at Malthus, 'neither war nor pestilence [had] a larger share perhaps than the prevailing modes of female dress',[53] for modern taste makes women pose and preen in skimpy cottons and muslins, 'half naked, all evening, braving disease and death', falling sacrificial victims 'in countless numbers, at the altar of fashion'.[54]

Fashion was generally judged one of the evils of modernity. Better, perhaps, to view it as a vestige of the savage state, equivalent to the tribesman's adoration of gaudy beads. And as a primitive force, this 'barbarous despotism of Fashion' tyrannized over commercial Britain no less than the Terror devastated revolutionary France:

> Their requisitions are as imperious as those of ROBESPIERRE, and as tamely endured. A table of diseases and of deaths, directly and indirectly produced by these requisitions, with the manner of their production . . . might be inscribed; THE REVENGE OF THE SLAVES OF REFINEMENT UPON THEIR TASKMASTERS.[55]

In fine, 'it seems impossible to live in the fret and fume of fashion without direct injury' to one's physique.[56] But it was not only in respect of attire that fashion exercised its evil sway. For the 'spoiled children of art' had now become addicted to proliferating artificial desires, wants, and needs – in a word, 'a new world of objects'. Enter consumer man. Indeed, judged Beddoes, 'it is upon an endless variety of ephemeral appendages to himself, to his retinue, or his mansion, that the heart of him who means to figure in the beau monde, is eternally set'. Yet such 'passion' was sick – in fact, 'more tormenting' even than the miser's 'thirst' for gold. The Timons of this world could at least store up 'solid and durable treasure'. But all was weariness, fever, and fret in the 'mart of the mode', for 'every new pattern makes all the old purchases worthless' – the result being that 'what these have cost creates a sense of vexation more violent, than a large stake, lost at the gaming table'.[57]

Thus fashion turned into a treadmill of disappointment and exhaustion for the 'I want it now' generation.[58] 'The multiplication of the roads to wealth unavoidably keeps pace with the multiplication of gratifications, and of those contrivances for displaying accomplishments, which wealth can command', argued Beddoes, 'for it is by profiting from the sale of these gratifications and these contrivances (that is, of the various luxuries of the table, of the toilet, of furniture, of equipage, of the fine arts) that more and more members of society grow rich.'[59] The outcome: running ever faster to stand still. Whereas 'savage life is uniform and dull', modern times had turned into a 'dance', a 'drama', an 'ever-moving picture'.[60] Yet all this furious flurry of fashion was no fun. The man of mode exhausts himself and ends up suffering a 'want of relish'.[61] 'The cells and conventicles of gentility . . . harbour beings, upon whose wearisome uniformity the tumult of pleasure never breaks in.'[62] Those attached to 'ephemeral appendages' and addicted to the 'rage for parties' are condemned to spicing up their dreary days with such 'provocatives' as alcohol and narcotics, 'that render the succeeding listlessness more intolerable, and another forced orgasm more indispensable'.[63]

In short, modern *moeurs* were a health danger, especially to the idle rich. 'Wealth exempts from certain kinds of labour. But the wealthy stretch this privilege a great deal too far for their good. . . . If we reckon from the middle station upwards, it would, I believe, be more just to assert, that the unhealthiness of families is in the direct, than that it is in the inverse proportion, of their wealth.'[64] After all, demanded Beddoes, 'does not gold bring with it its plagues?'[65] Those seduced by *la dolce vita* end up 'visited by the GOUT, the DROPSY, the PALSY – by the BLUE DEVILS, and OTHER COLOURED DEVILS lodged in the system'.[66]

The quintessential vice of the times, however, in Beddoes's eyes, was not mere greed, gluttony, or mindless acquisitiveness. It was the craving of the 'haves' to distinguish themselves over and above the 'have nots', through ever subtler refinements of life-style, ostentatious hallmarks of genteel superiority.[67] The escutcheon of politeness was sensibility. The pursuit of refinement meant abandoning the full-blooded active habits of ordinary tradesmen and craftsmen. After all, was not rude health *rude*, the birthmark of the *hoi polloi*? Such snobbery was an obvious recipe for sickliness.[68]

That conspicuous opulence 'which enables a greater proportion of the British to lead a life of comfort . . . than of the people of any other country', inevitably sapped the constitution of those 'who in shrinking from every comfortless sensation that may be occasioned by the action of the elements, are obliged to lead for a great part of the year a dusky chamber life. The foot that has always rested upon a carpet will be chilled if it tread upon a marble floor . . . at how much pains we have been to make ourselves too tender for the climate in which we live.'[69] Thus refinement enfeebled.

Delicacy, enervation ('relaxation' in the traditional sense of the term),[70] and even nervous sickliness were thus the brood of idleness – 'diseased sensibility is among the effects of long habituation to a high temperature in an atmosphere without motion'.[71] What appalled Beddoes was the fact that, through being such an evident emblem of fortune, sickliness had become a status symbol. Stuff and nonsense was being talked about 'the advantages of a feeble constitution', amid those selfsame smart circles parroting the modish humbug of Rousseau's 'disparagement of art and science'.[72]

Thus, Beddoes complains, modern mothers *à la mode*, anxious to hook a husband for their daughters, invest great effort into making them 'languid', lest one 'brought up with a sovereign regard to health, should not be delicate enough for the present demand'.[73] And the torture chamber *de rigueur* to render the daughters of the *nouveaux riches* sufficiently frail as votaries of the Graces was the boarding school. Cold, damp, stingy with rations, entirely without exercise facilities, and crushingly boring, the fashionable academy was guaranteed to make girls 'puny and drooping', or, as euphemism would have it, languid, delicate, and even terminally pretty[74] – for the modern academy 'has greatly contributed to multiply the genteel, linear consumptive make, now or lately so much in request'. It was all good for business: 'medical men have few better patrons' than proprietors of girls' schools.[75]

No surprise, then, that so many of the medical miseries of modernity 'have been laid to social refinement as its genuine but monstrous offspring'.[76] People cultivated an air of sensibility, but 'they find they have embraced sickliness instead of delicacy' – 'Alas for the abuse of terms,' Beddoes riposted: 'do we not hear the diseased perpetually styled *delicate*? Heaven knows how many this one *catachresis*, for that is the name of the said figure of speech, may have led to become candidates for disease, or at the least seduced into self-neglect.'[77]

Putting a stop to such absurd affectations was, however, no easy matter. Top people had to be persuaded to 'practise for improvement in health'.[78] The problem lay in convincing 'the ghastly beauties of the court and city' – those for whom 'the ruddiness of the milk-maid has been a standing jest'[79] – that robustness wasn't irremediably vulgar, even a 'curse'.[80] Direct means were bound to fail: health could not be sold to the *jeunesse d'orée* as natural or normal, still less as a duty. The answer lay, hinted the canny doctor, in fobbing it off as 'SOMEWHAT OF AN ACCOMPLISHMENT'.[81] Yet that could be but a start. 'The first great preservative of mental, as of bodily health, is active occupation'.[82] Unfortunately, affluence had rendered strenuous muscular activity appallingly uncouth.

Enlightenment and illness

Commercial civilization – with all its train of luxury, fashion, and refinement – thus hazarded the health of the affluent and aspirant. But equally deleterious was the mental culture gracing, or rather disgracing, this modish opulence: the Spectatorial ambience of the Enlightenment in its popularized forms. In smart society it had become essential to pass oneself off as witty, full of news, taste, opinions, and 'smart tripping chat' about faces and places, the latest ideas and events. Boorish Squire Westerns were out, polite accomplishments in. So the Quality were now bingeing on the books, rather as once they had on beefsteaks – and mental and moral indigestion was the inevitable sequela of 'cramming the head with dose after dose of heterogeneous ideas, before the first have had time to settle'.[83] Lives better given over to the field were being wasted on the sofa, eyes glued to duodecimos. And what were people the better for it? – Beddoes took a very dim view of this addling of the nation's brains by light reading in the names of amusement, instruction, and improvement: empty heads were being filled with vapid ideas.

Beddoes disapproved of the political hot-air literature of the time, advanced by 'second-rate reformers'.[84] Worse still were those terrible innovations, novels, which 'render the sensibility still more diseased': 'I cordially assent to the opinion of almost all men of reflection', thunders Beddoes, echoing Mrs Malaprop, that of all popular writing, 'NOVELS undoubtedly are the sort most injurious. . . . They increase indolence, the imaginary world indisposing those, who inhabit it in thought, to go abroad into the real.'[85] Novels fostered head-in-the-clouds fanta-sizing: 'The common love-stories are justly regarded as abominable. They relax soul and body at once' – and, Beddoes implies, though in the most mealy-mouthed terms, encourage teenage girls to masturbate.[86] Hopefully, things might change: 'As soon as science is a little more improved, and morals a little better understood, many admired novels will be banished in a body to the same shelf with Jack the Giant Killer and Tom Hickathrift.'[87]

More pernicious still, all this belletristic trash was now seeping down to children, for it was in an age in which 'parents overlay their young in blind fondness'.[88] Foolish ideals of genteel accomplishments had made schooling ever more bookish, and the specialist children's writer now hung out his shingle in Grub Street. Well-meaning though such authors might be, the genre was inevitably pernicious to physical and mental health, because the young should be exercising their muscles not their minds. 'The juvenile library!' he expostulated, 'with submission, I must consider it as little better than a repository of poisons. What acrimonies will it not engender in the habit! what obstructions in the body!'[89] Premature reading begat terrible maladies. 'The parent, when he brings a daughter or a son, "morbidly alive in every nerve", to the physician, should be candid enough to tell, how many dozens of Lilliputian volumes he devoured within a few years after he learned to read, and of how many hours' use of his limbs and sense he was daily defrauded in consequence.'[90] Ever faithful to the Rousseauvain pedagogics of his father-in-law, Richard Edgeworth, Beddoes insisted that we must 'render education less dependent upon books': otherwise the rising generation would grow up with crooked spirits and enfeebled shanks.[91]

In all such ways modern expectations, not least the march of mind, were making people sicker. Particularly disturbing was the fact that the spread of misguided polite intellectual culture also promoted wrong-headed ideas about maladies and medicine. If indiscriminate reading made people sick, their heads were also, in the process, being stuffed with a heteroclite mixture of simplistic and ill-digested medical maxims, culled from that very reading. The educated plumed themselves upon the notion that they understood their own health. Not so! 'Nothing is more fallacious than the common saying that every man of sense at forty knows what is good for his constitution.'[92]

Of course, the masses knew no better than to swear by their bits and pieces of medical magic, sayings, and saws. A little elementary psychology would explain how such dross implanted itself in their heads. An unthinking person might cut himself and start to bleed. Seeing the blood, the thought might flash into his mind that something red might help. Perhaps it worked, and so the magical idea of signatures and similars was born, and over the course of time, through the continuation of such primitive mental processes, 'the doctrine of diseases gradually puts on a more scholastic form'.[93] Once rooted, such ideas became almost indelible: 'it is wonderful with what avidity prejudices in physic as well as in religion are imbibed, and with what obstinacy they are retained by the untutored mind.'[94]

But such prejudices, Beddoes insisted, were not unique to yokels. In truth, 'medical superstition is to be sought, not only in the peasant's hut, but in the city and in the palace; beside the toilette of the lady of first fashion, and in the cabinet of the philosopher – more or less disguised perhaps, but still the same in substance'. Innumerable 'vulgar errors' were flying around, buoyed up by lay opinion.[95]

A sort of 'trickle down' process was at work, whereby, through books and gossip, professional medical arcana filtered into the public mind.[96] The trouble was that such ideas 'make their fortune in the world' only after being 'exploded' by science.[97] 'Opinions cast off, like threadbare apparel, by the faculty, go each in their turn to the public. *In the politest and best informed circles,* according to newspaper phraseology, no day probably passes without its victim to some antiquated hypothesis concerning the *purity of the blood, the acrimony of the juices, the transmigration of humours, the salubrity of the air of this or that spot.*'[98] Similarly with scrofula: everybody knew that the proper thing was to take scurvy grass, convinced that this would 'attenuate the humours, purify the blood or clear the passages' – but this was a worthless move, resting, Beddoes assured his readers, 'upon a wrong principle'.[99]

Thus tea-table chit-chat was riddled with 'erroneous domestic opinion'.[100] Some people insisted it would be a mistake to let scrofulous ulcers dry of, because, while running, they drained off peccant humours. Others had no doubt that if you dried up the tumour, the trouble would go away. Both were false.[101] And who knows how many bizarre ideas had accumulated around gout? Sufferers were, preposterously, pleased get a bout of gout, convinced that the disease protected them from more serious disorders. Totally absurd. Yet it was far from the only instance:

> In questions of medicine, the most obstinate belief is usually coupled with the most profound ignorance. What we hear uttered with oracular confidence, in sick apartments and at convivial meetings, over wine and round the tea-table, when it is considered as idle speculation, can only provoke a smile. But if it be regarded as, one day, destined to decide the fate of infants and of invalids, it must excite pity and horror.[102]

After all, Beddoes notes, the epidemic of hypochondria was proof enough of the power of all this claptrap. 'Some philosopher remarks, that a life would hardly suffice to enumerate the vain fantasies of mankind. No title in the list would, perhaps be more copious than that of suppositious and exaggerated diseases.'[103]

The smattering of pseudo-medical knowledge picked up and paraded by the laity produced one specially unfortunate outcome. It made lay people pose as infallible oracles upon doctors. Beddoes invites his readers to eavesdrop on a dialogue between a physician such as himself and a wiseacre patient, who has just rejected the services of a particular physician:

> 'But why?' you inquire, 'has *he* any marked deficiency of common sense?'
>
> 'Oh! As to common sense! I do not say that. But what is common sense! Is not something more wanted, where life itself is at stake?'
>
> 'True. In that I perfectly agree. But he has had, I am told, the usual opportunities for becoming thoroughly acquainted with his profession. Did he shew any particular negligence of disposition at the time of his studies? Or has he been a dissipated man since? Have you heard anything to that effect?'
>
> 'I cannot say I have. But this I know. For it came to me from one, who had it from a particular friend to the family. In my Lord Burroughdale's last illness, he certainly mistook a putrid for an inflammatory sore-throat; and had one ounce more of blood been taken, his lordship, I am confidently told, must have been rotten in his grave, by this time – Nay, the surgeon himself, it is whispered, hesitated about obeying the prescription for bleeding.'
>
> 'Such mistakes, sure enough, are far from pleasant.'
>
> 'Pleasant! what security have you against one as bad now? Such blunderers, really ought not – but I wonder how he ever got patients after my Lord's narrow escape'.
>
> 'Well, then, I thank you for your caution. And I believe I must call in Dr ——'
>
> 'What, Dr —— that notorious man of experiment, whom every body is crying out against! Did not he give iced water in a burning fever, though the whole world knows it is so hazardous to drink cold things, when hot? Nay, by carrying the prescription himself, my very next door neighbour discovered at the apothecary's, that he had ordered for his daughter arsenic, think of that! under a different name. Such a violent thing for such a poor puny creature as that girl! My God, and are human creatures then, not better than rats, that they are to be enticed to swallow poison in disguise!'
>
> 'I suppose then I send to Dr. F. Nothing like this can be alleged against him.'

> 'He! A mere Dr Slop. I'll answer for it, where something must be done without delay, you will as soon trust to your housekeeper's panada, as to Dr F.'s medicine.'[104]

'In this manner', concludes Beddoes, 'would a determined private practitioner traverse the whole list of graduates, English and Scotch. . . . His own recipe, he would still persevere in pressing as infallible.'[105]

'Private practitioner' was, Beddoes glossed, the in-term for a lay person who fancied his medical know-how. It was a scandalous imposition – 'what a winning thing is a genteel name' – no better than calling an assassin a 'private gentleman soldier'.[106] Such lay people – and the worst of them were the women, those 'busy-bodies in petticoats', said Beddoes in an aside, deploring 'the fatal authority of the sex in the medicine'[107] – felt no compunction about offering medical advice, forming diagnoses, and recommending medicines. Mixing 'self confidence and distrust of others',[108] 'these good people . . . have, strong upon them, the passion for snapping up verbal and written recipes for every current *name* of disease'. Some were 'public minded, and know no greater pleasure than in drawing from their magazine for the benefit of every acquaintance within reach of a call or a note';[109] others 'treasure up these stores for family use', taking pride in the charity that began at home: 'with what an air of satisfaction does one often hear it said; *we do such and such things within ourselves.* The phrase carries a happy union of economy, independence, security and mutual affection . . . what hedgehog, rolled up round, tight, and warm, in his skin, on a frosty morning, is more an object of envy than so close a family circle?'[110]

'Private practitioners' commonly trafficked in remedies. 'Numbers circulated scraps of paper, marked with medical hieroglyphics, just as they circulate scandal, for want of other employment',[111] and many such lay recipes acquired a spurious authority from being passed down in manuscript, having been 'originally transcribed from obsolete works, published during that barbarous state of pharmacy, from which this art has been of late much reclaimed. Of course, above ninety nine times in a hundred, practitioners of medicine have, in common use, improved formulas.' Here was yet further proof that new lay medicine was but bad old professional practice writ large.[112]

This proliferation of 'drugs in hands not taught their use' was specially scandalous.[113] 'Beware how you play the doctor's part',[114] Beddoes warned: was not ignorant dispensing equivalent to being 'turned blindfold into a apothecary's shop and giv[ing] your child the first drug you may lay your hands upon'? Imagine the shock, 'were a lady, educated and endowed as ladies usually are, to produce, from her pocket, a case of surgeon's instruments . . . nobody, I suppose, would submit to the hands of the operator'. For some silly reason, however, no one blanched at the thought of these lady doctors dishing out drugs by the dozen, 'the equally dangerous tools of the *physician*'.[115]

Drugging one's family, friends, and familiars could lead to serious consequences. It had become the done thing to dose oneself up with 'opiates in colds, whether as poppy syrup, or in the more fiery form of paregoric elixir, which is the base of many of our advertised cough drops. Whether disfigured, or prepared simply according to the college of physicians, the paregoric elixir has aggravated all the mischiefs which I have described as resulting from protracted colds.'[116] Not least, as Beddoes knew all too well from acquaintances such as Coleridge, self-administered opiates were the road to addiction.[117]

Overall, these 'private practitioners' were guilty of a mischievous 'kind of active personal imprudence (or disposition to interfere uncalled and unqualified) with the personal management of others)'.[118] By contrast to experienced regulars, the 'private practitioner' was at best like 'one rushing to the rescue in the dark'.[119] So why did they do it? Nothing but 'vanity' was 'the grand principle of this contraband trade', these adepts having an itch 'for being admired on account of trifles'.[120]

Yet the fault lay not entirely with the sick. For along with the 'private practitioner', Beddoes condemned the 'polite practitioner' too, for his eager collusion, for self-serving reasons, in the medical pretensions and presumptions of Quality patients.[121] One gross mercenary imposition of this kind was the publication, by regulars no less than by quacks and hacks, of handbooks of kitchen medicine and 'Every Man His Own Physician' manuals. Many of these, in particular the evergreen *Domestic Medicine* (1769) of William Buchan, quite openly justified the enterprise of 'laying physic open' before the people, by drawing upon the Enlightenment idiom of freedom and the rights of the people.[122]

Beddoes, who, of course, subscribed to such ideals in the political sphere, reckoned them inapplicable to medicine.

Consumers assumed a spurious medical expertise on the strength of owning such pestiferous volumes. They 'lay in a thick close-printed publication, purporting to be a family compendium of the practice of physic; then they place it, as shelf-companion to the bible, and hold it next in veneration to the sacred volume; the one being the fund from which they draw and dispense what is necessary to happiness in the life to come, the other in the present life'[123] (recall that Beddoes was, perhaps, in religion too an unbeliever). 'Certain adventurers' had undoubtedly 'obtained a degree of public confidence by their endeavours to popularize the practice of medicine'[124] – here Beddoes probably had Buchan in mind – but the truth was that a tome of domestic medicine was no less of a nonsense than one of teach-yourself shoe-making.[125] Medicine could not be learned from the circulating library: 'one has infinitely less chance of becoming an adept in medical matters without regular study, than of becoming rich without regular industry.'[126]

People revered such tomes as treasure troves of wisdom, investing them with unwarranted confidence: 'if there were safety in the multitude of books', Beddoes chaffed, 'parents would have little to apprehend for their progeny. The literature of Europe abounds with productions on the diseases and the management of children.'[127] In reality, however, society was being bombarded with junk reading. 'I may, I believe,' Beddoes commented, 'presume upon it as a pretty generally allowed fact, that in no line is there so large a proportion of bad hands as in that of book-making . . . none in which the wholesale vendors more frequently contrive to pass worthless articles upon the consumer.'[128] Not a single worthwhile work of domestic medicine existed – 'I doubt whether any physician of avowedly large experience . . . has ever undertaken to instruct the unprepared public, in the general knowledge and treatment of disorders.'[129] And a bad book of home physic was bound to be 'productive of disastrous consequences'.[130]

The road to reform

The *literati* and the *glitterati* thus made rods for their own backs. They pursued sickly life-styles; they set misplaced confidence in their own medical skills; and, not least, by corrupting their medical attendants, they sapped the salubrious power of physic.

Their fault? – They wanted it both ways. 'A child is ridiculed for thinking that he can eat his cake and have it. Are not grown people equally ridiculous, if they complain of ailments at the time they are doing every thing in their power to bring them on? – There can be no hope of avoiding them, unless we be filled by a *sentiment* of the value of health, at least as lively as that which animates us to the pursuit of any other temporal blessing. . . . Whoever', concludes Beddoes, perhaps with a blush, 'can inspire the public with this sentiment will do more good than the discoverer of twenty specific remedies.' Things had to change.[131]

For one thing, the public needed to learn not to mess with medicine. Every churchyard showed the 'fatal effects, arising from domestic errors'.[132] Keep off! He warned, for

> Persons out of the profession incur too great a risk, and I wish they could be made to feel more responsibility, when they meddle with the administration of medicines. If they think it too much to call in a physician on every *slight* occasion, they may change this opinion in some degree, if they consider that they must be very imperfect judges concerning occasions, and that a physician, acting with success on seeming slight occasions, will render his unavailing assiduities in emergencies less frequently required. So that there will be a certain economy of the person, and a probable one of the purse.[133]

But Beddoes was far from wholly negative. Fatalism was not in order. Rousseau may have judged the 'state of nature' the 'sole preventive for the diseases of society', but his was a wayward and wilful pessimism. True, curative medicine had far to go, 'the imperfection of the healing art being an incontestible fact, to which not only every bill of mortality, but every assemblage of gravestones bears witness'.[134] But there could be no going back: 'to accelerate the progress of civilization is probably our only practical and only effectual plan.' No time for nostalgia or hand-wringing,

> it may, at least, be worth while to consider, whether the exertion of intellect cannot repair mischiefs, which it must be allowed to have incidentally produced, and whether that havoc of health and life, with which our civilization is

> justly upbraided, may not be the effect of the barbarism which it still retains in its composition.[135]

Thus further progress must be the answer to the problems of progress. The lesson of health will not come spontaneously – 'it must, no doubt, be taught' – but, eventually 'consciousness of health, thus contemplated, will become just as much a source of pleasure as consciousness of virtue'.[136]

To effect such improvements, researchers must advance medical science, and clinicians deploy it in treating disease. So what were the public to do? Their lot lay not with 'remedying' disorders but with 'preventing' them – for 'prevention is better than cure'.[137] They should look to 'preservation' not 'restoration'.[138] The people thereby had an active, prophylactic role in health, for they should acquaint themselves with the 'diseases of society'[139] and join in anticipating them. Yet prevention – though a 'great and precious . . . art' – was currently 'neglected'.[140] Hence Beddoes aimed to persuade his readers to pursue 'habitual well-being'[141] and thereby health, that 'first of blessings'.[142] Blinded by the glamour of medicine, people had almost forgotten the meaning of health, to say nothing of its value:

> 'What is good against the head-ache, Doctor?' 'Health, Madam.' 'Well, if you feel no interest about an old woman like me – Marianne there, you perceive, has been hacking all the afternoon. Do tell her of some little thing, that is good against a cough.' 'Health, Madam.' 'But are you resolved not to give a more satisfactory answer? In that case, I shall take the liberty of guessing why.' 'Poh! Mrs W. ——', cried a grave person in spectacles, from behind a full hand of cards – 'you should know that it is the trick of these gentlemen NEVER TO SPEAK PLAIN, as some great man says. And if they will not in a tete-a-tete, can you expect it before company?' 'I am not conscious of having uttered any enigma. I am sorry for the young lady. But I must still answer – health, Sir, health, Madam'.[143]

'The lady', Beddoes concludes, 'it will appear from the preceding little fragment, belongs to the corps, from which I am ambitious to enlist recruits.'[144]

The laity should not trespass upon the practitioner's vocation of combating sickness: its task was to safeguard its health. In the fulfilment of this duty, doctors could help. Beddoes, as we have seen, wanted to expose and reform the pathological habits of high society. But he also sought to instruct readers in the basic laws of hygiene. Indispensable to that end was increased attention to the body, its laws, and its needs. Indifference and prudery had to be broken down.[145] 'The exterior of the human body', Beddoes reflected, 'is frequently contemplated with the highest delight and but seldom, in its healthy state, with disgust.' By contrast, there was little 'familiarity with the internal parts', and unfortunately, thanks to our 'customs, it requires an exemption to overcome the repugnance which arises on observing them attentively for the first time'. (The stomach, confesses the fat physician, 'in man and in animals resembling man is far from recommending itself by any elegance of appearance'.)[146]

To this end, Beddoes proposed courses of anatomical and physiological lectures for the public, women included, and also, more daringly, open clinical lectures, involving demonstrations upon volunteer 'indigent sufferers'.[147] Anticipating opposition, he explained:

> I do not see why popular CLINICAL lectures should not be joined to popular anatomical lectures. . . . It must be their aim to make fully sensible the mischiefs arising from systematic irregularity; from injudicious management after exposure to the inclemencies of the weather, and from the other innumerable ordinary errors of individual conduct. They must explain the origin and conduct, much more minutely than the treatment of diseases. They may be conveniently undertaken wherever there exists an infirmary.[148]

Such demonstrations would help secure the happiness of posterity 'in the most effectual manner'.[149]

Above all, children had to be given instruction, to 'distinguish the parts of the body. Such information will lead them to observe many important changes, which as they take place slowly, are apt to proceed unobserved.' If only the young were capable of describing their ills more accurately, early diagnosis would improve in diseases such as scrofula.[150] This applied not just to children. 'The ignorant of all denominations, and the poor and the young amongst the rest, we perpetually find unable to fix, with any tolerable accuracy, the seat of their maladies. Hence arises one great difficulty in their treatment.'[151] How stupid of society to teach the 'anatomy and physiology of external prosperity', while ignoring the welfare of people's very bodies: 'The very same reason that makes it advantageous to be able, at the shortest warning, to call before us a summary of our *pecuniary* circumstances, applies with at least equal force to our *personal* circumstances.'[152]

Of course, there would be obstacles. Advocating setting up 'in every one of our considerable towns, lectures for a *mixed* audience, on select subjects of ANATOMY', Beddoes feared such a proposal would be deemed unEnglish, and

> innumerable mothers, though accustomed to consider themselves but as instruments for promoting the well-being of their offspring, will feel an unconquerable repugnance against paying any sort of attention to our internal conformation, even though the means of instruction be placed ever so conveniently within their reach. That we are *fearfully and wonderfully made* they will piously believe, but every particular proof of this proposition they will consider as lying beyond their province.[153]

How absurd that those itching to meddle with medicines should disdain truly to advance health.[154]

In short, it was crucial that the public acquire a knowledge of the 'laws of their own existence' and the 'science of the human structure and functions'.[155] Thereby 'physiology will come to be considered as the domestic science *par excellence*'.[156] His own writings were offered as one step in that direction, containing not a word about home medicine or surgery, but being entirely devoted to 'applying physiological knowledge to domestic uses'.[157]

Beddoes deplored such public blindspots. Fashionable people neglected their health, but loved playing the doctor. The public enthusiastically patronized Humane Societies for resuscitating the drowned, but hardly gave a thought – or a penny – to the infinitely larger numbers of tuberculosis victims – 100,000 a year, he guessed.[158] Though living among 'legislators equally unacquainted with the subject of national health',[159] Beddoes aimed to launch campaigns of health education and action. Would not some noble lord become a patron of public health, rather as the Duke of Bedford had supported husbandry? The Government had established a Board of Agriculture, why not a Board of Health? Surely enlightened and philanthropic industrialists, now setting up dispensaries and infirmaries among their work-forces, would enlarge their activities and do their bit for prevention at their works. And above all, Beddoes sought an educational drive, 'education, in the enlarged, proper sense of that term', whose first goal would be to dispel error:

> So much is there to unlearn on the present subject, that to reduce the mind to that *blank* state in which, according to Locke, it originally exists, would be no mean advantage to four out of five among those, who may take up these essays. The author is certainly accustomed to see invalids, for whom it would be happy if their whole mass of ideas – provided those were included that relate to the means of their recovery – could be abolished. No physician but must have found disorders less difficult to manage than patients, and both disorders and patients together, less difficult than the friends of patients.[160]

Having thus wiped the slate clean, the health educator could at last reform the patient, by laying bare the social sources of sickness, and by instructing the people, not in physic, but in health. It would be a long haul, but it was possible. If, at the dawn of the French Revolution, Beddoes had waxed messianic about the imminent revolution in medicine, by the 1800s, when tackling popular health education, his tone was more sombre, sardonic, self-mocking even. Thanks to his own and his colleagues' writings, he notes, children were now enjoying a better diet: 'and so happy a change is probably an indication that strong public and private remonstrances from medical men, if they be continued half a century, will have a real influence on the condition of their fellow creatures.'[161]

Conclusion

Such self-deflating irony contains the heart of the matter. Beddoes hoped that he, as a doctor, as an educator, as a writer, as a man of Enlightenment, could promote a solution. He was also sufficiently self-aware that he might be part of the problem. After all, his own profession had to shoulder much of the blame for the parlous perversions of medical practice, for it was practitioners who condoned any nonsense the laity wanted to believe. Illness was business. It was, after all, his profession that was profiteering hand-over-fist from such obscene temples to Moloch as watering-places.[162] After all, the spirit of the Enlightenment – as expounded by William Buchan's *Domestic Medicine* (1769) and his followers, commonly called the 'Buchaneers' – was for putting medicine in lay hands. After all, he was himself, a prolific writer of tomes targeted at the public. If authorship were perhaps a counter-productive activity, if popular addiction to reading was a health risk, could Beddoes – writing books against bookishness, in a manner mirroring the paradoxes of Burton and Sterne – himself escape censure with a good conscience? ('Will this be good for your worship's eyes?') Beddoes was not, I believe, unaware of the ironies of his own self-created situation.[163]

In the end, the cause of reforming the patient hinged upon education. Would it work? Was it even a consistent, credible option? Everyone wanted to teach, no one to learn. 'There is a foible, even more common among the instructors of little people, than among us authors, who pretend to instruct the large public. Both take much greater pleasure in giving than in following good advice. Both would rather find faults in others, than amend their own.'[164] Wasn't doling out more opinions to the opinionated liable to prove self-defeating?

Beddoes devoted a couple of hundred pages of the *Hygeia* – that work of 'moral materia medica' – to savaging the system of public schools for boys (which prized 'emulation [and] confinement',[165] neither a very estimable quality) and boarding schools for girls. Affording no education, such establishments merely ruined morals and health alike. All the same, he never wavered from his vision – derived explicitly from Locke and Hartley – of human beings as essentially educable creatures. And that meant all folks – not least the lower orders, and even domestic nursemaids ('It is by no means so impracticable as many would fain make us believe, to eradicate . . . prejudices from the minds of female attendants'). All minds were much of a muchness – 'there is much less disparity in the power of apprehension of different ranks, than the superior members of society are willing to flatter themselves'.[166] What was crucial was the right method of teaching – 'it can very seldom be done by threats or by commands'; maids could be given, not orders, but explanations, 'without derogation from authority'.[167]

If people were, finally, capable of learning through experience, explanation of their present parlous state of ignorance, superstition, and misinformation was, nevertheless, no simple task. But there were at least grounds for hope and certainly scope for improvement.

This chapter, it goes without saying, has not been claiming that we hear, recorded in Thomas Beddoes's writings, the authentic voice of *fin-de-siècle* high society, drawling its own vulgar errors. Beddoes, it is true, may be credited with paying attention to his patients, and with having a good ear. He clearly believed that a good physician must be a good listener – though it was a much-neglected skill: 'a great cloud is left upon the powers of most substances, employed in medicine, because physicians have been at little pains to record the history of patients, subsequent to their recovery.'[168] Beddoes wanted this to change:

> When I meet with invalids observant of themselves and disposed to communicate, it has long been my custom to request a particular narrative, in writing of all the circumstances which they suppose to have any relation to their complaint. It is the only way, I believe, to get at the knowledge of the original causes of disorders when they lie in any way remote.[169]

The sick person's story was the Ariadne's thread. He praised a 'patient whose journal of his illness seems to me to give a clearer representation of the ebbs and flows and eddies of the mind in epilepsy, than all the writings of medical men put together'.[170] If this was, indeed, an era in which, as medical historians tell us, physicians were becoming less disposed to listen to their patients, these reflections are worth bearing in mind.

All the same, the voice of the sick as recorded in Beddoes's advice literature is obviously a construct, a fiction, and one deftly crafted to suit Beddoes's own strategic purposes. As a meritocratic medical scientist, he needed to forge myths of lay meddlesomeness – all those dreadful petticoat doctresses! – as a foil to his future vision of unchallenged professional authority. Yet as a radical and populist, Beddoes was eager not to silence the people but to reform them, changing them from would-be Aesculapians into devotees of Hygeia. It is this vision of the future lay role – active, health-conscious as a person, passive, compliant as a patient – which Beddoes's thinking promotes. Scholars of the nineteenth century have yet to tell us how far Beddoes's prescription – dream or nightmare – actually came about.[171]

Notes

1. For this standard view, see F. F. Cartwright, *A Social History of Medicine* (London: Longman, 1977). For the broader politics of reform, see Asa Briggs, *The Age of Improvement, 1783–1867* (London: Longman, 1959). My thanks to Andrew Wear and Christine Stevenson for their Beddoesian criticisms.

2. Ivan Waddington in particular has argued that contemporary medical reforms essentially shored up the *status quo*: 'The struggle to reform the Royal College of Physicians, 1767–1771: a sociological analysis', *Medical History*, 17 (1973), 107–26; 'The role of the hospital in the development of modern medicine: a sociological analysis', *Sociology*, 7 (1973), 211–24; 'The development of medical ethics – a sociological analysis', *Medical History*, 19 (1975), 36–51; 'General practitioners and consultants in early nineteenth century England: the sociology of an intra-professional conflict', in J. Woodward and D. Richards (eds), *Health Care and Popular Medicine in Nineteenth Century England: Essays in the Social History of Medicine* (London: Croom Helm, 1977), pp. 164–88; *The Medical Profession in the Industrial Revolution* (Dublin: Gill & Macmillan, 1984).

3. For such writings, see Waddington (references given in note 2); S. W. F. Holloway, 'Medical education in England, 1830–1858: a sociological analysis', *History*, 49 (1964) 299–32; I. S. L. Loudon, 'The origin of the general practitioner' (The James Mackenzie Lecture of the Royal College of General Practitioners for 1982), *Journal of the Royal College of General Practice*, 33 (1983), 13–18; I. S. L. Loudon, 'The nature of provincial medical practice in eighteenth-century England', *Medical History*, 29 (1985), 1–32; I. S. L. Loudon, "The Vile Race of Quacks With Which This Country is Infested"', in W. F. Bynum and Roy Porter (eds), *Medical Fringe and Medical Orthodoxy, 1750–1850* (London: Croom Helm, 1987), pp. 106–28; I. S. L. Loudon, *Medical Care and the General Practitioner 1750–1850* (Oxford: Clarendon Press, 1986).

4. N. Jewson, 'Medical knowledge and the patronage system in eighteenth century England', *Sociology*, 8 (1974), 369–85; N. Jewson, 'The disappearance of the sick man from medical cosmology, 1770–1870', *Sociology*, 10 (1976), 225–44.

5. H. Brody, *Stories of Sickness* (New Haven: Yale University Press, 1987); A. Kleinman, *The Illness Narratives: Suffering, Healing ad the Human Condition* (New York: Basic Books, 1988); E. J. Cassel, *Talking to Patients* (Cambridge, Mass.: MIT Press, 1985); L. M. Beier, *Sufferers and Healers: The Experience of Illness in Seventeenth-Century England* (London: Routledge & Kegan Paul, 1987); Roy Porter, 'The patient's view: doing medical history from below', *Theory and Society*, 14 (1985), 175–98; Roy Porter (ed.), *Patients and Practitioners: Lay Perceptions of Medicine in Pre-Industrial Society* (Cambridge: Cambridge University Press, 1985).

6. M. Foucault, *The Birth of the Clinic*, trans. A. M. Sheridan Smith (London: Tavistock, 1973).

7. M. E. Fissell, 'The physic of charity: health and welfare in the West Country, 1690–1834', University of Pennsylvania, PhD thesis, 1988.

8. For Beddoes's career, see J. E. Stock, *Memoirs of the Life of Thomas Beddoes MD* (London: J. Murray, 1811); D. A. Stansfield, *Thomas Beddoes M.D. 1760–1808, Chemist, Physician, Democrat* (Lancaster: Reidel, 1984); F. F. Cartwright, 'The association of Thomas Beddoes, M.D. with James Watt, F.R.S', *Notes and Records of the Royal Society of London*, 22, (1967) 1 & 2, 131–43; F. W. Gibbs and W. Smeaton, 'Thomas Beddoes at Oxford', *Ambix (9 February 1961), xx–xx;* L. S. Gottlieb, 'Thomas Beddoes M.D. and the Pneumatic Institution at Clifton 1798–1801', *Annals of Internal Medicine*, 530–3; T. H. Levere, 'Dr Thomas Beddoes at Oxford, radical politics in 1788–93, and the fate of the Regius Chair in Chemistry', *Ambix*, 28, 2 (July 1981), 61–69; T. H. Levere, 'Dr Thomas Beddoes and the establishment of his Pneumatic Institution: a tale of three presidents', *Notes and Records of the Royal Society of London*, 32 (1977), 41–9; T. H. Levere, 'Thomas Beddoes, the interaction of pneumatic and preventative medicine with chemistry', *Interdisciplinary Science Review*, 7, (1982) 137–47; A. Miller, 'The Pneumatic Institution of Thomas Beddoes at Bristol', *Annals of Medical History*, New York, 1931.

9. Important among Beddoes's publications are *A Letter to Erasmus Darwin . . . on a new method of treating pulmonary consumption, and some other diseases hitherto found incurable* (Bristol: Bulgin & Rosser, 1793); *Considerations on the Medicinal Use of Factitious Airs and on the manner of obtaining them in large quantities. Part I by Thomas Beddoes (Part II by James Watt)*, 1st edn (Bristol: Bulgin & Rosser; London: J. Johnson, 1794); *A Lecture Introductory to a Course of Popular Instruction on the Constitution and Management of the Human Body* (Bristol: Joseph Cottle, 1797); *Essay on the Causes, Early Signs, and Prevention of Pulmonary Consumption for the use of parents and preceptors* (Bristol: Biggs & Cottle, 1799; 2nd edn, London: Longman & Rees, 1799); *Observations on the medical and domestic management of the consumptive; on the powers of digitalis purpurea; and on the cure of scrophula* (London: Longman, 1801); *Hygëia: or essays moral and medical, on the causes affecting the personal state of our middling*

and affluent classes, 3 vols (Bristol: J. Mills, 1802); *Manual of Health: or, the Invalid conducted safely through the seasons* (London: Johnson, 1806); *A Letter to the Right Honourable Sir Joseph Banks . . . on the causes and removal of the prevailing discontents, imperfections, and abuses, in medicine* (London: Richard Phillips, 1808).

10. For further details, see Roy Porter, 'The people's health in Georgian England', to appear in T. Harris (ed.), *Popular Culture* (London: Macmillan, 1991). Beddoes detested Hannah More, repeatedly – in his private correspondence with Davies Giddy – calling her 'hypocritical'. Yet he had no doubt that it was the job of the middle class to reform the poor, and was paid the rather ambiguous compliment of being asked, by Miss More's supporters, for permission to reprint his tract against drunkenness, *The History of Isaac Jenkins, and of the sickness of Sarah his wife, and their three children* (Madeley 1792). This book was indeed reissued several times in the nineteenth century by do-gooders.

11. Beddoes, *Hygëia: or essays moral and medical, on the causes affecting the personal state of our middling and affluent classes*, 3 vols (Bristol: J. Mills, 1802–3).

12. Beddoes, *Manual of Health: or, the Invalid conducted safely through the seasons* (London: Johnson, 1806).

13. Beddoes, *Hygeia*, vol. 1, essay i, p. 8. (further references will appear in the form 1 i 8).

14. Beddoes, *Hygeia*, 1 i 9.

15. For Beddoes and the shortcomings of regulars, see Roy Porter, 'Plutus or Hygeia? Thomas Beddoes and medical ethics', in R. Baker, D. Porter, and R. Porter (eds), *The Codification of Medical Morality in the Eighteenth and Nineteenth Centuries*, vol. 1, (Dordrecht: Kluwer, 1991), xx–xxx.

16. For Beddoes on quacks, see Roy Porter, *Health for Sale: Quackery in England 1660–1850* (Manchester: Manchester University Press, 1989), pp. 199–202.

17. For a characterization of the Enlightenment in England, see Roy Porter, 'The Enlightenment in England', in Roy Porter and Mikulas Teich (eds), *The Enlightenment in National Context* (Cambridge: Cambridge University Press, 1981), pp. 1–18; Roy Porter, 'Was there a medical Enlightenment in eighteenth century England?', *British Journal for Eighteenth Century Studies*, 5 (1982), 46–63; Seamus Deane, *The French Revolution and Enlightenment in England 1789–1832* (Cambridge, Mass.: Harvard University Press, 1989).

18. For Beddoes's optimism, see Roy Porter, 'Thomas Beddoes and the advancement of science', unpublished paper; Roy Porter, 'Medicine in the Enlightenment', in E. Mendelsohn (ed.), *Enlightenment, Science and Ideology* (Cambridge, Mass.: Harvard University Press, 1990).

19. Beddoes, *Hygeia*, 2 vii 98. For contemporary epidemiology, see M. J. Dobson, 'Population, disease and mortality in Southeast England, 1600–1800', DPhil thesis, University of Oxford, 1982; M. J. Dobson, 'A chronology of epidemic disease and mortality in Southeast England, 1601–1800', *Historical Research Series*, 19 (1987); M. J. Dobson,

From Old England to New England: Changing Patterns of Mortality (Oxford: School of Geography University of Oxford Research Paper 38, 1987); U. Tröhler, 'Quantification in British medicine and surgery 1750–1830; with special reference to its introduction into therapeutics', PhD thesis, University of London, 1978.

20. Roy Porter, 'Plutus or Hygeia? Thomas Beddoes and medical ethics', in R. Baker, Dorothy Porter and Roy Porter (eds), *The Codification of Medical Morality in the Eighteenth and Nineteenth Centuries*, vol. 1, (Dordrecht: Kluwer, 1991), xx–xxx.

21. Beddoes, *Hygeia*, 1 i 46; Beddoes, *A Letter to the Right Honourable Sir Joseph Banks . . . on the causes and removal of the prevailing discontents, imperfections, and abuses, in medicine* (London: Richard Phillips, 1808), pp. 97, 100.

22. Beddoes, *Hygeia*, 1 i 9. For eighteenth-century views of the perverting effects of commerce, see J. G. A. Pocock *Virtue, Commerce and History* (Cambridge: Cambridge University Press, 1985); John Sekora, *Luxury: The Concept in Western Thought, Eden to Smollett* (Baltimore: Johns Hopkins University Press, 1977). For contemporary perceptions of the relations between the march of civilization and growing threats to health, see Roy Porter, 'Commerce and disease in eighteenth century England', in P. G. Bouce (ed.), *Ideology in Eighteenth Century England* (Paris: forthcoming). For today's sociological debate, see also D. Miller, *Material Culture and Mass Consumption* (Oxford: Basil Blackwell, 1987).

23. Beddoes, *Hygeia*, 1 ii 52.

24. Beddoes, *Hygeia*, 1 iii 11.

25. For these views, see Roy Porter and Mikulas Teich (eds), *The Enlightenment in National Context* (Cambridge: Cambridge University Press, 1981); John Brewer and Roy Porter (eds), *Consumption and the World of Goods* (London: Routledge, 1990). See Beddoes, *Hygeia*, 1 iii 81: 'British consumers are supplied not only by British producers but the labourers of almost every other country administer to the sensuality or to the indolence of our richer classes.'

26. Beddoes, *Hygeia*, 1 iii 6 and 10. On rival prophecies in the 1790s, see Seamus Deane, *The French Revolution and Enlightenment in England 1789–1832* (Cambridge, Mass.: Harvard University Press, 1989).

27. Beddoes, *Hygeia*, 1 iii 84. See also Roy Porter 'Consumption in the consumer society', in John Brewer and Roy Porter (eds), *Consumption and the World of Goods* (London: Routledge, 1990). See also T. Beddoes, *A new method of treating pulmonary consumption* (xx, xx, 1794); Beddoes, *Essay on the Causes, Early Signs, and Prevention of Pulmonary Consumption for the use of parents and preceptors* (Bristol: Biggs & Cottle, 1799; 2nd edn, London: Longman & Rees, 1799).

28. Beddoes, *Manual*, 143, 135.

29. Beddoes, *Hygeia*, 2 viii 91. Bristolians were proverbially money-grubbing. See M. Neve, 'Natural philosophy, medicine and the culture of science in provincial England: the cases of Bristol, 1796–1850 and Bath, 1750–1820', PhD thesis, University of London, 1984; J. Barry, 'The cultural life of Bristol, 1640–1775', DPhil thesis, Oxford University, 1986.

30. Beddoes, *Hygeia*, 3 x 77.
31. Beddoes, *Hygeia*, 3 x 77.
32. This felicitous phrase is due to C. B. Macpherson.
33. Beddoes, *Hygeia*, 1 iv 29. On credit, see John Brewer, 'Commercialization and politics', in N. McKendrick, John Brewer, and J. H. Plumb, *The Birth of a Consumer Society: The Commercialization of Eighteenth-Century England* (London: Europa, 1982), pp. 197–264; Julian Hoppit, 'The use and abuse of credit in eighteenth century England', in N. McKendrick and R. B. Outhwaite (eds), *Business Life and Public Policy* (Cambridge: Cambridge University Press, 1986).
34. Beddoes, *Hygeia*, 1 ii 71.
35. Beddoes, *Hygeia*, 1 ii 72.
36. Beddoes, *Hygeia*, 1 ii 52.
37. Beddoes, *Hygeia*, 1 ii 58 and 60.
38. Beddoes, *Hygeia*, 1 ii 57 and 58.
39. Beddoes, *Hygeia*, 3 ix 207. Such views had earlier been expounded by George Cheyne. See the introduction by Roy Porter to G. Cheyne, *The English Malady* (London: Routledge Reprint, 1990; 1st edn, 1734).
40. Beddoes, *Hygeia*, 3 ix 207.
41. Beddoes, *Manual*, 33.
42. Beddoes, *Manual*, 131.
43. See Pocock, *Virtue, Commerce and History*; Sekora, *Luxury*; Porter, 'Plutus or Hygeia?'.
44. On the differences between Cheyne's and Beddoes's critiques, see the introduction by Roy Porter to G. Cheyne, *The English Malady* (London: Routledge Reprint, 1990; 1st edn, 1734).
45. Beddoes, *Hygeia*, 1 ii 64; see also Roy Porter, 'The language of medicine in eighteenth century England', in Peter Burke and Roy Porter (eds), *Words, Words, Words* (Cambridge: Polity Press, 1990).
46. Beddoes, *Manual*, 307. For the implications of polite language, see Roy Porter, 'The language of medicine in eighteenth century England', in Peter Burke and Roy Porter (eds), *Words, Words, Words* (Cambridge: Polity Press, 1990).
47. Beddoes, *Hygeia*, 2 v 60.
48. Beddoes, *Hygeia*, 3 ix 163. '*Hypocrite auteur, mon semblable, mon frère*', one is tempted to respond.
49. Beddoes, *Hygeia*, 1 ii 65.
50. Beddoes, *Hygeia*, 2 vii 99. For the eighteenth-century child treated as a consumer object and status symbol, see Linda Pollock, *Forgotten Children: Parent–Child Relations from 1500 to 1900* (Cambridge: Cambridge University Press, 1983); Linda Pollock, *A Lasting Relationship: Parents and Children over Three Centuries* (London: Fourth Estate, 1987); J. H. Plumb, 'The new world of children in eighteenth-century England', *Past and Present*, 67 (1975).
51. Beddoes, *Hygeia*, 1 ii 62. Compare the Bath physician and writer, J. M. Adair, *Essays on Fashionable Diseases* . . . (London: Bateman, 1790): (p. 1) 'fashion like its companion Luxury, may be considered as one of those excrescences which are attached to national improvement'; (p. 2) 'As societies advance in civilization, the

active mind of man, not contented with the means of satisfying our natural wants, is anxiously employed in creating artificial wants, and inventing the means of their gratification'; (p. 2) 'the empire of fashion has now become universal; it is not confined to the decorations of our persons, or the embellishment of our houses and equipages; but extends to our politics, morals, religion, and even in some degree to our sciences. Men and women of fashion are supereminently distinguished from those of no fashion, or whom, no-body knows.' For discussion, see A. Forty, *Objects of Desire: Design and Society 1750–1980* (London: Thames & Hudson, 1986).

52. Beddoes, *Hygeia*, 1 ii 81 and 71.

53. Beddoes, *Hygeia*, 1 iii 75 and ii 71.

54. Beddoes, *Hygeia*, 1 iii 74.

55. Beddoes, *Hygeia*, 1 ii 73, 75–6.

56. Beddoes, *Hygeia*, 1 ii 70.

57. Beddoes, *Manual*, 163; *Hygeia*, 1 ii 70. For extensive discussion of consumption and the meaning of things, see N. McKendrick, John Brewer and J. H. Plumb, *The Birth of a Consumer Society: The Commercialization of Eighteenth-Century England* (London: Europa, 1982); John Brewer and Roy Porter (eds), *The Origins of the Consumer Society* (London: Routledge, 1990); Lorna Weatherill, *Consumer Behaviour and Material Culture, 1660–1760* (London: Routledge, 1988); Lorna Weatherill, 'Consumer behavior and social status in England', *Continuity and Change*, 2 (1986), 191–216; Lorna Weatherill, 'A possession of one's own: women and consumer behaviour in England, 1660–1740', *Journal of British Studies*, 25 (1986), 131–56; A. O. Hirschman, *The Passions and the Interests; Political Arguments for Capitalism before its Triumph* (Princeton: Princeton University Press, 1977).

58. Beddoes, *Hygeia*, 1 ii 52.

59. Beddoes, *Hygeia*, 1 ii 53.

60. Beddoes, *Hygeia*, 1 ii 53 and 54. This acceleration of life is well conveyed by F. D. Klingender, *Art and the Industrial Revolution*, ed. A. Elton (St Albans: Paladin, 1968).

61. Beddoes, *Hygeia*, 1 ii 62.

62. Beddoes, *Hygeia*, 1 ii 62.

63. Beddoes, *Hygeia*, 1 ii 70. 'Orgasm' here does not have a narrowly sexual meaning. See also 1 ii 65; 1 ii 62, and for the wider problem of alcohol and addiction, see the introduction by Roy Porter to Thomas Trotter, *An Essay on Drunkenness* (London: Routledge Reprint, 1989; 1st edn, 1804); Thomas Trotter, *A View of the Nervous Temperament* (London: Longman, Hurst, Rees & Owen, 1807), p. 105.

64. Beddoes, *Hygeia*, 1 ii 54.

65. Beddoes, *Hygeia*, 1 ii 57.

66. Beddoes, *Hygeia*, 1 ii 57.

67. On the growing separation of élite and popular culture, see Pierre Bourdieu, *Distinction: A Social Critique of the Judgement of Taste* (Cambridge, Mass.: Harvard University Press, 1984); J. M. Golby and A. W. Purdue, *The Civilization of the Crowd: Popular Culture in England, 1750–1900* (London: Batsford, 1984); Peter Burke, *Popular Culture in*

Early Modern Europe (London: Temple Smith, 1978); R. Malcolmson, *Popular Recreations in English Society 1700–1850* (Cambridge: Cambridge University Press, 1973).

68. Janet Todd, *Sensibility, An Introduction* (London: Methuen, 1986).

69. Beddoes, *Manual*, 132.

70. Roy Porter and Dorothy Porter, *In Sickness and in Health: The British Experience, 1650–1850* (London: Fourth Estate, 1988), chs 2 and 3.

71. Beddoes, *Manual*, 134.

72. Beddoes, *Manual*, 3.

73. Beddoes, *Hygeia*, 1 iii 62.

74. Beddoes, *Manual*, 214, 233.

75. Beddoes, *Hygeia*, 1 iii 12.

76. Beddoes, *Hygeia*, 1 i 87.

77. Beddoes, *Hygeia*, 1 iii 63; *Manual*, 17.

78. Beddoes, *Manual*, 21.

79. Beddoes, *Manual*, 14.

80. Beddoes, *Manual*, 7.

81. Beddoes, *Manual*, 7.

82. Beddoes, *Hygeia*, 3 x 79.

83. Beddoes, *Hygeia*, 1 iii 32.

84. Beddoes, *Hygeia*, 1 iii 78. In the 1790s, Beddoes was a fiery radical. I do not believe his radicalism ever diminished. His expectations of rapid and imminent political improvement did not, however, last beyond about 1795. He became a very disappointed man.

85. Beddoes, *Hygeia*, 1 iii 77.

86. Beddoes, *Hygeia*, 1 iii 78. On masturbation, see P.-G Bouce, 'Les Jeux interdits de l'imaginaire: onanism et culpabilisation sexuelle aux XVIIIe siècle', in J. Céard (ed.), *La Folie et le corps* (Paris, Presses de l'Ecole Normale Supérieure, 1985), pp. 223–43; E.H. Hare, 'Masturbatory insanity: the history of an idea', *Journal of Mental Science*, 108 (1962), 1–25; R. H. MacDonald, 'The frightful consequences of onanism', *Journal of the History of Ideas*, 28 (1967), 423–41; J. Stengers and A. Van Neck, *Histoire d'une grande peur: la masturbation* (Brussels: University of Brussels Press, 1984); L.J. Jordanova, 'The popularisation of medicine: Tissot on onanism', *Textual Practice*, 1 (1987), 68–80.

87. Beddoes, *Hygeia*, 1 iii 78.

88. Beddoes, *Manual*, 38.

89. Beddoes, *Hygeia*, 3 ix 166.

90. Beddoes, *Hygeia*, 3 ix 167. On Edgeworth, see W. A. C. Stewart and W. A. McCann, *The Educational Innovators, 1750–1880* (xx, xx, 1967).

91. Beddoes, *Hygeia*, 3 ix 169. D. Clarke, *The Ingenious Mr Edgeworth* (London: Oldbourne, 1965).

92. Beddoes, *Hygeia*, 2 viii 54.

93. Beddoes, *Hygeia*, 1 i 50.

94. Beddoes, *Hygeia*, 1 i 51.

95. Beddoes, *Hygeia*, 2 vi 64.

96. See N. McKendrick, John Brewer and J. H. Plumb, *The Birth of*

Consumer Society: The Commercialization of Eighteenth-Century England (London: Europa, 1982); John Brewer and Roy Porter (eds), *The Origins of the Consumer Society* (London: Routledge, 1990).

97. Beddoes, *Hygeia,* 1 i 51 and 52.

98. Beddoes, *Hygeia,* 1 i 52. For lengthier discussion, see Roy Porter, 'The people's health in Georgian England', to appear in T. Harris (ed.), *Popular Culture* (London: Macmillan, 1991); and Dorothy Porter and Roy Porter, *Patient's Progress: Doctors and Doctoring in Eighteenth Century England* (Stanford: Stanford University Press, 1989; Cambridge: Polity Press, 1989), ch. 11.

99. Beddoes, *Hygeia,* 2 vi 66.

100. Beddoes, *Hygeia,* 2 vi 64.

101. Beddoes, *Hygeia,* 2 vi 72.

102. Beddoes, *Hygeia,* 1 i 45; 1 i 48. For the spread of lay opinion, see Dorothy Porter and Roy Porter, *Patient's Progress: Doctors and Doctoring in Eighteenth Century England* (Stanford: Stanford University Press, 1989; Cambridge: Polity Press, 1989), ch. 3.

103. Beddoes, *Hygeia,* 1 i 58; on hypochondria, see E. Fischer-Homberger, 'Hypochondriasis of the eighteenth century – neurosis of the present century', *Bulletin of the History of Medicine,* 46 (1972), 391–401; S. Baur, *Hypochondria: Woeful Imaginings* (Princeton: Princeton University Press, 1988).

104. Beddoes, *Hygeia,* 1 ii 23.

105. Beddoes, *Hygeia,* 1 ii 25.

106. Beddoes, *Hygeia,* 1 ii 20. Cf. J. M. Adair, *Essays on Fashionable Diseases* . . . (London: Bateman, 1790), p. 73, with its condemnation of 'the empiricism of lady and gentleman doctors'.

107. T. Beddoes, *A Letter to the Right Honourable Sir Joseph Banks . . . on the causes and removal of the prevailing discontents, imperfections, and abuses, in medicine* (London: Richard Phillips, 1808), p. 113.

108. Beddoes, *Hygeia,* 1 ii 22.

109. Beddoes, *Hygeia,* 1 ii 16.

110. Beddoes, *Hygeia,* 1 ii 17; see also Dorothy Porter and Roy Porter, *Patient's Progress: Doctors and Doctoring in Eighteenth Century England* (Stanford: Stanford University Press, 1989; Cambridge: Polity Press, 1989), ch. 3.

111. Beddoes, *Hygeia,* 1 ii 29.

112. Beddoes, *Hygeia,* 1 ii 29.

113. Beddoes, *Hygeia,* 1 ii 22.

114. Beddoes, *Hygeia,* 2 vii 94.

115. Beddoes, *Hygeia,* 1 ii 40 and 38.

116. Beddoes, *Manual,* 197.

117. Roy Porter and Dorothy Porter, *In Sickness and in Health: The British Experience, 1650–1850* (London: Fourth Estate, 1988), ch. 11; V. Berridge and G. Edwards, *Opium and the People* (London: Allen Lane, 1981); N. Fruman, *Coleridge, the Damaged Archangel* (London: Allen & Unwin, 1971).

118. Beddoes, *Hygeia,* 1 ii 40.

119. Beddoes, *Hygeia,* 1 ii 46.

120. Beddoes, *Hygeia*, 1 ii 27.

121. Beddoes, *Manual*, 358; Roy Porter, 'Plutus or Hygeia? Thomas Beddoes and medical ethics', in R. Baker, D. Porter and R. Porter (eds), *The History of Medical Ethics* (Dordrecht: Reidel, 1991).

122. Roy Porter, 'The patient in eighteenth century England', in A. Wear (ed.), *History of Medicine in Society* (Cambridge: Cambridge University Press, forthcoming); see also Roy Porter, 'The people's health in Georgian England', in T. Harris (ed.), *Popular Culture in the Eighteenth Century* (London: Macmillan, 1991).

123. Beddoes, *Hygeia*, 1 ii 18.

124. Beddoes, *Hygeia*, 1 ii 33.

125. Beddoes, *Hygeia*, 1 ii 19; C. Lawrence, 'William Buchan: medicine laid open', *Medical History*, 19 (1975), 20–35; C. Rosenberg, 'Medical text and medical context; explaining William Buchan's *Domestic Medicine*', *Bulletin of the History of Medicine*, 57 (1983), 22–4.

126. Beddoes, *Hygeia*, 1 ii 15. For Beddoes's extremely demanding notion of a proper medical education, see Roy Porter, 'Plutus or Hygeia? Thomas Beddoes and medical ethics', in R. Baker, Dorothy Porter and Roy Porter (eds), *The History of Medical Ethics: The Eighteenth Century* (Dordrecht: Reidel, 1991).

127. Beddoes, *Hygeia*, 2 v 6.

128. Beddoes, *Hygeia*, 1 ii 18.

129. Beddoes, *Hygeia*, 1 ii 31.

130. Beddoes, *Hygeia*, 1 ii 19.

131. Beddoes, *Hygeia*, 1 iv 97.

132. Beddoes, *Hygeia*, 3 xi 92.

133. Beddoes, *Manual*, 193.

134. Beddoes, *Hygeia*, 1 ii 33.

135. Beddoes, *Hygeia*, 1 i 89.

136. Beddoes, *Hygeia*, 1 i 84.

137. Beddoes, *Manual*, 200.

138. Beddoes, *Manual*, 32.

139. Beddoes, *Hygeia*, 1 i 88.

140. Beddoes, *Hygeia*, 3 xi 86.

141. Beddoes, *Hygeia*, 1 i 16.

142. Beddoes, *Hygeia*, 1 i 16.

143. Beddoes, *Hygeia*, 1 ii 14 and 15.

144. Beddoes, *Hygeia*, 1 ii 15.

145. Beddoes, *Hygeia*, 2 viii 6.

146. Beddoes, *Hygeia*, 2 viii 7.

147. Beddoes, *Hygeia*, 2 vi 92.

148. Beddoes, *Hygeia*, 2 vi 91.

149. Beddoes, *Hygeia*, 2 vi 91.

150. Beddoes, *Hygeia*, 2 vi 46.

151. Beddoes, *Hygeia*, 2 vi 47.

152. Beddoes, *Hygeia*, 1 i 29.

153. Beddoes, *Hygeia*, 1 i 37 and 39.

154. Beddoes, *Hygeia*, 1 i 40. Beddoes gave such lectures, which were apparently a success [MSS].

155. Beddoes, *Hygeia*, 1 i 34; 36.

156. Beddoes, *Hygeia*, 2 vi 48.
157. Beddoes, *Hygeia*, 1 i 54.
158. Beddoes, *Hygeia*, 3 xi 3.
159. Beddoes, *Hygeia*, 1 ii 81.
160. Beddoes, *Hygeia*, 1 i 53. For further details, see Roy Porter, 'Thomas Beddoes and the advancement of science', unpublished paper.
161. Beddoes, *Hygeia*, 1 iii 28.
162. Roy Porter, 'Get a smart sea-sickness if you can: travelling for health in eighteenth century England'.
163. L. Sterne, *The Life and Opinions of Tristram Shandy*, ed. C. Ricks (Harmondsworth: Penguin, 1967), p. 265. See also Roy Porter, 'Against the spleen', in V. G. Myer (ed.), *Laurence Sterne: Riddles and Mysteries* (London and New York: Vision Press, 1984), pp. 84–99.
164. Beddoes, *Hygeia*, 1 iii 15.
165. Beddoes, *Hygeia*, 1 iii 59.
166. Beddoes, *Hygeia*, 2 v 16.
167. Beddoes, *Hygeia*, 2 v 16. For the psychological background, see J. Yolton, *John Locke and the Way of Ideas* (Oxford: Oxford University Press, 1956); J. Yolton, Thinking Matter (Minneapolis: Minneapolis University Press, 1984); Robert M. Young, 'Association of ideas', in P.P. Wiener (ed.), *Dictionary of the History of Ideas*, 4 vols (New York: Scribner's Sons, 1973).
168. Beddoes, *Hygeia*, 2 viii 127.
169. Beddoes, *Hygeia*, 2 vii 9.
170. Beddoes, *Hygeia*, 3 ix 33.
171. For some doubts as to whether the nineteenth century saw much change in the conduct of the sick, see Roy Porter and Dorothy Porter, *In Sickness and in Health: The British Experience, 1650–1860* (London: Fourth Estate, 1988); Roy Porter and Dorothy Porter, *Patient's Progress: Doctors and Doctoring in Eighteenth Century England* (Stanford: Stanford University Press, 1989; Cambridge: Polity Press, 1989).

2

Private enterprise and public interests: medical education and the Apothecaries' Act, 1780–1825[1]

Susan C. Lawrence

The Apothecaries' Act of 1815 stands as a signpost within the history of medical education and the medical profession in Britain. As the first parliamentary enactment to require licensing by examination for a large number of medical men – all those who intended to give medical advice and to dispense medicines throughout England and Wales – it marks the watershed between the heyday of unregulated (although not necessarily unqualified) practitioners and the rise of increasing state supervision over entry into the medical profession. Whether the signpost pointed forwards, towards a better educated, respectable general practitioner, or backwards, confirming the apothecary's subservience to the physician and shackling him to the indignities of apprenticeship, has been a much argued point.

Smug practitioners and complacent historians eulogized the Act as progressive legislation in a reforming era, leading to a near revolution in medical education as schools sprang up to provide the courses the Apothecaries' Act demanded and hospitals opened their wards for required clinical instruction.[2] The Act's contemporary and modern critics, in contrast, bemoaned its limited scope, as the regulations touched neither the élite physicians and surgeons, whose London colleges continued to supervise their qualifications, nor lowly chemists and druggists, commonly believed to be encroaching on respectable practice from their shops. By requiring apprenticeship and initially demanding only a narrow range of medical courses, moreover, the Apothecaries' Act appeared to confirm the traditional tripartite structure of the British medical profession, hindering the development of a unified occupation which recognized the general practitioner's essential role in an industrializing society.[3] The Act was, in short, a flawed compromise in which servility coexisted uneasily with regulatory responsibility.

Most of the discussion about the Act's origin and effects has been based on three types of sources. First, the diverse and scattered collection of medical periodicals, pamphlets, and petitions provides the reformers' rhetoric, which emphasized the threatening hordes of unqualified practitioners. Second, the minute books of the Royal Colleges and the Society of Apothecaries contain the official pronouncements of educational policies, which uniformly reveal that the traditional bastions of the tripartite profession in London held on to their privileges and conservatism in the face of reform. Finally, the 1834 Report of the Select Committee on Medical Education (SCME) offers a wealth of testimony from practitioners about medical education and practice from those involved with the Act's conception or administration, much of it, however, understandably given with either congratulatory or critical hindsight.[4] These sources are invaluable for their insight into the public controversy surrounding the Act and the opinions that many medical men had of its impact. They lack, nevertheless, specific evidence on how the Act affected aspiring practitioners in its early years and insight into the more subtle ways that it shaped medical education. Further archival material, notably the Society of Apothecaries' registration books, which listed each candidate's qualifications upon examination, can illuminate these issues.[5]

A quantitative analysis of the candidates' applications for the Apothecaries' licence (the LSA) during the Act's first four years offers a useful perspective from which to view the development of medical education in England. Tabular annual snapshots constructed from these data reveal both the relatively high qualifications of the first applicants and the initial changes in the candidates' formal medical education. The data from these first years are intelligible only if they are seen in light of the cumulative effect of long-term changes in medical teaching. Indeed, the Apothecaries' assumptions about necessary course work and clinical experience arose directly from the thriving – and unregulated – system of private medical education in London. As the candidates' certificates demonstrate, moreover, the London hospitals and dispensaries competed to provide the required months of clinical instruction. The metropolis unquestionably appears as the major British centre for the education of general practitioners.

The figures from later years further indicate that the Apothecaries' Act, by solidifying contemporary expectations and upholding a nearly unquestioned procedure of licensing by corporate examination, helped to entrench a bureaucratic process inherited from traditional medical institutions. While reform debates continued with undiminished fervour into the nineteenth century, few challenged the structure established as the Society of Apothecaries successfully carried out its duties: a central body of examiners who set educational standards, demanded proof of compliance from their applicants and certified practitioners after a short examination. By the late 1820s and early 1830s, the Society subtly began to use the authority it had over its candidates to regulate medical education more precisely, determining the appropriate number of lectures in a 'course', for example, and defining what they would accept as a 'hospital'. Looking at the day-to-day decisions the Apothecaries made in determining educational criteria and in examining candidates suggests that such mundane procedures increasingly led the examiners to circumscribe, although not to circumvent, the 'free-market' model of medical education that dominated London teaching in the first half of the nineteenth century.[6]

The Apothecaries' Act thus undoubtedly highlights a major transition in British medical education: the shift from haphazard, individualistic and unregulated instruction to a standardized, monitored, and required series of courses and clinical practice for non-university medical men. Both the absence of regulations certifying 'legitimate' medical men outside London and the wide variations in acceptable and available medical education before the Act made the Society's licence mandatory for 'professional' apothecaries have made it difficult to assess reformers' claims that England teemed with unqualified practitioners. During the eighteenth century, just about anyone could, in fact, compound and dispense medicines, perform surgery, and deliver infants, although with little legal recourse for recovering fees for such services. In London, neither the Corporation of Surgeons (in 1800 the Royal College of Surgeons) nor the Society of Apothecaries, outside the City, had an effective monopoly over practice. The Royal College of Physicians technically could prosecute non-members who charged for medical advice within a seven-mile radius of the City, but the nuisance and expense of going to court meant that the College rarely invoked this privilege.[7]

Training for those who provided medical care for the vast majority of the population ranged from *ad hoc* experience picked up by clergymen, farmers, and part-time midwives to years of formal instruction at Edinburgh or Leyden. Throughout the 1700s, nevertheless, many full-time practitioners, who did not initially aim to gain MDs and hence to practise as physicians, acquired their education through a combination of apprenticeship, taking courses at private homes or lecture theatres, and walking the wards of a London or provincial hospital. Apprenticeship was the time-honoured route to the apothecary's trade and the surgeon's craft and survived well into the nineteenth century. While formally structured by the apprentice's indenture, which specified that the master would prepare his pupil for his occupation, the apprentice's opportunities varied widely in practice. Certainly no regulations outlined either the content or the level of expertise the young man should acquire. Parental, community, and cultural expectations, in addition to the master's concern for his reputation, sufficed to ensure that the apprentice was duly bred to care for the sick.[8]

Gradually emerging over the eighteenth century, however, post-apprenticeship education through lectures and hospital experience developed under the initiative of scores of men who sold extra knowledge and expertise for modest fees. London's teaching entrepreneurs catered especially to a crowd of aspiring practitioners who could not afford the time or expense of a university degree. From a handful of courses in the first decades of the century, London lecturers and the London hospitals' physicians and surgeons offered an increasing number of courses and opportunities for clinical work that not only rivalled university programmes, particularly those at Edinburgh, but also were extremely flexible and relatively inexpensive. This unstructured system especially appealed to aspiring apothecaries, surgeons, and the popular hybrid, the surgeon-apothecary-man-midwife.[9]

In the autumn of 1800, for example, London lecturers advertised five courses in anatomy, five in chemistry and materia medica, eight in midwifery, seven in the theory and practice of medicine, four in the theory and practice of surgery, three on practical anatomy (dissection), and three sets of clinical lectures. In addition, all of the seven general hospitals – St. Thomas's, Guy's, St. Bartholomew's, the London, St. George's, the Middlesex and the Westminster – had short-term paying pupils walking their wards in growing numbers. By the first years of the nineteenth century, at least 300 students a year signed up to observe hospital practice, most of them following the surgeons on their rounds.[10] Surviving student accounts suggest that young men tailored their London work to supplement the knowledge and skills acquired in apprenticeship. Richard Kay, an apothecary's pupil at Guy's in 1743–4, chose to hear lectures on anatomy, surgery, and midwifery in preparation for his intended career as 'both Surgeon and Physician' in Lancashire. In 1812–13, John Green Crosse, surgeons' pupil at St. George's, not only took courses in anatomy and surgery, clearly in line with his early ambition to become a 'pure' surgeon, but also attended lectures in chemistry, medicine, and midwifery after his provincial apprenticeship.[11]

As the Corporation/Royal College of Surgeons and the Society of Apothecaries neither required nor particularly encouraged formal lecture courses or hospital experience for membership before the early nineteenth century, the steady growth of London's diverse medical curricula reflects a direct response to a cultural shift in Georgian society: the demand for 'middling' rank, respectable practitioners who could make a comfortable, but not spectacular, living from medicine. For young men seeking to enhance their professional and social status, a stay in the metropolis was likely to be well worth the expense. The 'academic' courses, the drama of ward rounds, the lure of the theatre and popular preachers may well have given some practitioners subtle advantages for breaking into the competitive market for patients. The sheer number of medical courses advertised year after year between 1770 and 1815, moreover, suggests that scores of unlicensed medical men were as 'qualified' for practice, according to contemporary expectations, as official members of the three London corporations.

Into this voluntary system, established and thriving on private enterprise, came the late-eighteenth- and early-nineteenth-century calls to reform the medical profession and to eliminate competition from druggists, irregulars, and other 'unqualified' medical attendants. Those whose own standards had been raised by years in Edinburgh or London sought to establish minimum requirements for all *bona fide* medical men, ideally through joint examinations for surgeons and apothecaries or, even better, a separate college or examining board, while leaving the certification of 'pure' physicians and surgeons to the Royal Colleges, even though their jurisdiction was limited to London. The rhetoric of reform was full of appeals to the public interest: the poor and the ignorant, as well as the rich and knowledgeable, would benefit from a closed profession, whose leaders could monitor entry and prosecute unlicensed practitioners.

The resultant Apothecaries' Act, which Parliament passed on 11 July 1815, required that apothecaries then entering practice throughout England and Wales hold their licence, and as such was a minor victory for those hoping to curtail irregular practice. That it excluded chemists and druggists, who were left unlicensed, and kept medical qualifications distinct from surgical ones, immediately frustrated those hoping for more powerful and comprehensive legislation.[12] Whatever disappointment reformers felt when faced with the Act's final form, however, power over *de facto* general practitioners had been granted to the Society of Apothecaries, whose recent concerns had lain much more with its role as a City trading company than with that as a licensing corporation.[13] When George Man Burrows, a leading reformer and member of the Society, was asked to join the twelve-member Court of Examiners in July 1815, he was dismayed to discover that several of his colleagues 'did not know such an Act was in existence'.[14] Despite their apparent uninterest, the Court proceeded to decide on educational criteria, organize publication of the new regulations, establish remuneration for the examiners, and prepare forms with which to receive the expected influx of candidates when the Act went into effect on 1 August 1815.[15]

The Apothecaries' initial educational provisions were hardly innovative. The Act allowed the Court of Examiners to establish whatever qualifications they thought necessary for examination, although technically they could not dispense with the mandatory five-year apprenticeship, which was written into the Act itself. In July 1815, the examiners drew up a list of preliminary rules. In addition to evidence of apprenticeship, the candidate was to produce testimonials of good moral character, of having taken six three-month courses (two in anatomy and physiology, two in the theory and practice of medicine, one in chemistry, and one in materia medica), and of having followed six months' medical practice at a hospital, dispensary, or infirmary.

By 1815, apprenticeship, course work, and hospital practice

were already well-established routes for preparing for a respectable medical career, although some already argued that apprenticeship was outmoded, menial, and unscientific.[16] As stressed above, many private lecturers in London offered the courses the examiners required, either in extramural rooms or at four of the general hospitals. At about three to four guineas a session (five to six guineas for dissection courses in anatomy), a student could fulfil the Apothecaries' lecture requirements for between twenty and twenty-six guineas.[17] Both London and provincial hospitals had long allowed ward-walking students, while fragmentary evidence suggests that dispensary physicians and surgeons in London had begun to profit from a few pupils who observed their out-patient practices.[18] In principle, therefore, the Apothecaries' examiners did no more than codify an educational pattern familiar in London. They extended what those who could afford extra-apprenticeship work had voluntarily chosen to all young men seeking to become apothecaries or general practitioners.

Like the Royal College of Surgeons and the Royal College of Physicians, moreover, the Society of Apothecaries acted simply as a licensing body for the candidates. From the foundation of these corporations, entry had rested upon fulfilling criteria to become a candidate, an examination, and a fee. After their split from the Barber-Surgeons in 1745, the Surgeons' Corporation dropped their apprenticeship requirement, relying almost exclusively upon an oral examination for their military certificates and general diplomas until 1810. From this time, the Royal College of Surgeons' examiners began to expect proof that a candidate had taken courses and seen some hospital practice. The Royal College of Physicians demanded a valid MD degree of its applicants for the licentiate, limiting the fellowship almost exclusively to graduates of Oxford or Cambridge, followed by an oral examination.[19] Neither group had a mechanism beyond the actual examination for assessing the content or extent of their candidates' previous education. At this stage, therefore, the Society of Apothecaries mirrored its fellow corporations by setting specific educational criteria in the public's interest, while presuming that private – and unregulated – lecturers and institutions would provide the means for students to fulfil these requirements. The Society neither certified instructors nor monitored course content nor inspected hospitals, dispensaries, and infirmaries for their level of clinical instruction. For the first ten years of the Act, private enterprise flourished, with lecturers and institutions hotly competing to provide the services which the examiners demanded.[20]

While it is now abundantly clear that the Apothecaries' Act did not create either medical lectures or clinical instruction in London or the provinces, little attention has focused on its administration or immediate effect. As the Apothecaries' first hundreds of candidates sweated out their examinations, the Society began to face the tensions inherent in a system that gave them public responsibility for certifying practitioners whose background qualifications rested on testimonials of apprenticeship, course work, and clinical experience which were still private and unregulated. Delving into the minutiae of the Apothecaries' examinations allows at least a partial reconstruction of the examiners' tasks and reveals the range of the candidates' qualifications, London's dominance in medical instruction, and portents for the Society's later, more elaborate regulations.

To evaluate the Act's initial impact on medical education as revealed by the Society's registration books, it is important to consider first the extent and validity of the data they provide. When a candidate appeared for examination, a clerk filled out a form, checking off the testimonials, indentures, course tickets, and certificates which the student was required to bring to verify his background (see Table 2.1). In most cases, the clerk noted the name of the student's principal examiner and the outcome, passed or rejected.[21] These forms thus offer information on a candidate's apprenticeship, the number – although not the location – of the courses taken, and where he observed medical practice. There are certain seductive dangers, however, in taking this evidence entirely at face value. First, clerks make mistakes; how many or of what kind is impossible to estimate.[22] Second, the form has no room to note courses taken in other than the required subjects, such as midwifery or the theory and practice of surgery, and hence probably under-represents the breadth of pupils' education. Third, it is possible that students brought only enough certificates to satisfy the minimum requirements and hence did not register the full extent of their courses or training.[23] It is unlikely, nevertheless, that most of these 'marginal' students did so, given the pressure to establish credibility in front of the examiners.[24] Whether the extent of training is under-reported, moreover, is not crucially significant: the data from the registers presented the Apothecaries'

Table 2.1 Form used to enter the applicant's qualifications at Apothecaries' Hall, 1 August 1815–31 July 1817

181

MR. CANDIDATE FOR A
CERTIFICATE TO PRACTICE AS AN APOTHECARY IN
AN APPRENTICE TO MR.
APOTHECARY for Years.

TESTIMONIAL FROM

LECTURES

COURSES ON ANATOMY AND PHYSIOLOGY
_______ THEORY AND PRACTICE OF MEDICINE
_______ CHEMISTRY
_______ MATERIA MEDICA

HOSPITAL ATTENDANCE

MONTHS AT
as

MONTHS AT

examiners with the *apparent* calibre of their applicants, which would have influenced their judgement on the efficacy of their standards.

The Apothecaries' Act went into effect on 1 August 1815; the examiners saw their first candidate ten days later. Between this date and 31 July 1819, 865 men applied for a licence.[25] Table 2.2 presents an overview of the applicants. The number of applicants nearly doubled in four years, which suggests the pressing need among general practitioners for the privilege of dispensing medicines. Over 90 per cent regularly passed; in the spring and summer of 1818–19, the clerk unfortunately became careless and did not note outcomes on many of the forms. According to the Society's figures given to the Select Committee on Medical Education, in that year 94 per cent passed.[26] The average failure rate for this period was nearly 5 per cent. Most students applied for a licence to practise in the country, defined as outside a ten-mile radius around the City, rather than a London certificate.[27] Finally, 60–4 per cent of the students had filled the minimum of five years' apprenticeship, with a small –

Table 2.2 Apothecaries' candidates: 1815–19

	1815–16		*1816–17*		*1817–18*		*1818–19*	
Candidates	190		184		221		270	
Passed	173	91%	171	93%	209	95%	169	63%
Failed	16	8%	6	3%	10	4%	12	4%
Unknown	1		7	4%	2	1%	89	33%
Certificates for								
Country	174	92%	167	91%	209	95%	235	87%
London	15	8%	17	9%	12	5%	15	5%
Unknown	1						20	7%
Apprenticed for								
< 5 years	9	5%	3	2%	2	1%	6	2%
5 years	114	60%	118	64%	139	63%	175	65%
6 years	16	8%	23	12%	28	13%	29	11%
7 years	47	25%	38	21%	50	23%	57	21%
> 7 years	4	2%	2	2%	2	1%	3	1%

yet significant – number of applicants having less than this. Several longer-term students applied for the licence before their indentures had expired. The examiners recognized years served, rather than completed apprenticeships, as an adequate preparation for practice.

The general figures, while showing the magnitude of the examiners' tasks, hide the range of their judgements on who could be admitted to the examinations. When broken down according to the Society's technical criteria, the data show that the examiners had considerable flexibility in awarding their licences (see Table 2.3). An average of 9 per cent of the candidates were passed *without* the necessary course work, hospital experience, or (more rarely) apprenticeship. In a few of these cases the decision was inexplicable; in others, it reveals the examiners' realistic understanding that other work made the student adequately qualified. During the first year, for example, four men who had served in the army or navy, all of whom produced evidence of five years' apprenticeship, were passed without having taken any courses at all.[28] Others demonstrated personal knowledge apparently acquired from private study. William Barker, for example, who registered on 24 October 1816, had completed five years' study at the Manchester

Table 2.3 Apothecaries' candidates: 1815–19: marginal and over-qualified applicants

	1815–16		*1816–17*		*1817–18*		*1818–19*	
Candidates	190		184		221		270	
Number *passed* without the minimum qualifications	19	10%	18	10%	21	9%	17	6%
Number *failed/ unknown* without the minimum qualifications	5	3%	1		4	2%	15	6%
Number submitting the exact course and practice requirements	*8*	*4%*	*24*	*13%*	*38*	*17%*	*56*	*21%*
Marginal applicants	32	17%	43	23%	63	28%	88	33%
Over-qualified applicants	158	83%	141	77%	158	72%	182	67%

Infirmary, which he submitted as fulfilling the requirements for both apprenticeship and clinical practice. While he had evidence of only three courses in anatomy and physiology, the clerk noted that he 'has prepared almost all the preparations of the Pharmacopoeia'. Such attainments admitted him to the examination, where he passed without needing evidence of having taken courses in medicine, chemistry, or the materia medica. The examiners' willingness to consider officially 'unqualified' candidates, therefore, did not reflect simply lax standards, but rather demonstrates their flexibility when faced with unusual, but competent, candidates.[29]

The assumption that the examiners simply shut their eyes, bent their rules, and licensed poorly qualified men became one of the publicized criticisms of the Act's administration. On 25 March 1817, George Man Burrows resigned from the Court of Examiners in part due to the way the Court had handled an unqualified candidate in October 1816. In this instance, as Burrows explained at length to the public in his 1817 *A Statement of the Circumstances Connected with the Apothecaries' Act and its Administration*, the applicant had been apprenticed to a druggist and chemist, not to a recognized apothecary as required. The student's admission to examination, which he passed, established a dangerous precedent, as well as flouting the law. Yet Burrows's resignation appears to have come from his continued dissatisfaction with the examiners and their close, stultifying links with the Court of Assistants that impinged upon the examiners' independence. From his own account, Burrows was also a stickler for formality, objecting, for example, to verbal instead of written contact with the Court of Assistants, and held deep disappointments with the Act that the Society refused to address. His long-held frustration with the Court exacerbated the circumstances surrounding his dissent over the qualifications of this particular candidate. Burrows did not mention or dispute the significant number of other young men who had already obtained their LSAs improperly, although he generally bemoaned the poor showing many candidates made in examinations.[30] Burrows's hard line, therefore, over the applicant apprenticed to the druggist and chemist must be balanced with the other examiners' initial common-sense acceptance of contemporary standards for ordinary medical practitioners.

While the pass rate for technically unqualified students remained fairly high during these years, the number who submitted evidence of having the exact minimum of courses and practice rose considerably, from 4 per cent to 21 per cent. The obverse of this growth is perhaps more telling: the number of over-qualified applicants (those with more courses or longer practice) declined from 83 per cent to 67 per cent. As noted above, this drop may simply reflect how some students chose to register. These figures nevertheless suggest that, while the Act broadened the educational standards for the pool of aspiring apothecaries, at the same time it narrowed the higher range of qualifications that many students were pursuing when the Act was implemented: more students chose to get by with less work.

A more refined analysis reveals how the applicants' range of qualifications shrank during the Act's first four years, particularly in the courses taken and the practice seen (see Table 2.4). Overall, the average number of courses which candidates took dropped steadily from 8.4 in 1815–16 to 7.8 in 1818–19.

Table 2.4 Apothecaries' candidates: 1815–19: number of courses taken

	1815–16		*1816–17*		*1817–18*		*1818–19*	
Candidates	190		184		221		270	
Course averages								
Anatomy (2)	2.87		2.26		2.46		2.48	
Medicine (2)	2.23		2.28		2.20		2.15	
Chemistry (1)	1.89		1.88		1.75		1.70	
Materia Medica (1)	*1.29*		*1.39*		*1.46*		*1.50*	
Total average	8.39		8.21		7.87		7.83	
Course totals								
< 6 courses	16	8%	15	8%	20	9%	22	8%
= 6 courses	46	25%	50	27%	63	29%	73	27%
> 6 courses	73	38%	78	42%	96	43%	132	49%
> = 10 courses	55	29%	41	22%	42	19%	43	16%

Fewer students took extra courses in anatomy, the theory and practice of medicine, and chemistry, while more added lectures on the materia medica. Examining the distribution of the total number of courses registered reveals, furthermore, a considerable decline in the percentage of pupils who took ten or more courses, from 29 per cent in 1815–16 to 16 per cent in 1818–19. Here are clear signs of the narrowing of qualifications towards the middle range, slightly above the minimum required for licensing.

Similarly, the length of clinical practice seen at a hospital, dispensary, or infirmary shifted towards the minimum between 1815 and 1819. As Table 2.5 shows, in 1815–16, 34 per cent of the applicants submitted evidence of having attended two medical institutions or different practices within the same hospital, and 64 per cent of these visits lasted more than six months. By 1818–19, only 4 per cent registered with certificates for more than one practice, and a mere 21 per cent of these attendances lasted more than six months.

Some students may well have sat the Apothecaries' examination as soon as they finished the minimum requirements, perhaps to budget time in case they failed and needed to repeat the test. With the Society's licence in hand, they could then have gone on to take more courses and to complete a year as a

Table 2.5 Apothecaries' candidates: 1815–19: duration of medical practice at hospitals, dispensaries, and infirmaries

	1815–16		*1816–17*		*1817–18*		*1818–19*	
Candidates	190		184		221		270	
Evidence for								
one practice	125		156		197		258	
two practices	65 (34%)		27 (15%)		24 (11%)		12 (4%)	
Total entries	255		210		245		282	
Duration								
< 6 months	4	2%	5	2%	6	2%	10	3%
= 6 months	82	32%	77	37%	127	64%	210	75%
6-12 months	133	52%	91	43%	36	15%	32	11%
> 12 months	30	12%	30	14%	44	18%	28	10%

surgeons' pupil in order to qualify for membership in the Royal College of Surgeons. The overwhelming impression on the Apothecaries' examiners, nevertheless, must have been the appearance of a decided decline in students' initiative and qualifications in the years immediately after the Act went into effect.

The registers reveal other trends which were probably of less concern to the Apothecaries' examiners, but are of undoubted interest to historians. In 1968, Sir Zachary Cope praised the influence of the Apothecaries' Act in improving medical education, particularly emphasizing the examiners' demand for clinical instruction in a hospital, dispensary, or infirmary. Cope (and others) have argued that dispensaries especially filled the demand for practical medical experience with patients that hospitals apparently did not provide.[31] In contrast, Irvine Loudon has recently argued, after analysing the Apothecaries' SCME data from 1832–4, that 'the dispensaries never played a major part in medical education.'[32] Tracking the candidates' choices of clinical experience suggests that both of these strong generalizations are partially correct and highlights how competing institutions first responded to the examiners' provisions.

During the first year of the Act, 80 per cent of the applicants presented evidence that they had followed practitioners on the wards of one of the general London hospitals: St. Thomas's, St. Bartholomew's, Guy's, the Westminster, St. George's, the

London, or the Middlesex (see Figure 2.1).[33] London dispensaries, provincial hospitals and dispensaries, Scottish medical institutions – primarily the Edinburgh Royal Infirmary – and military experience account for the rest. Of the candidates who went to the London hospitals, however, only about 18 per cent specified that they had followed the physicians or apothecaries on rounds. Forty-three per cent had attended the surgeons, while for 38 per cent the type of practice was not filled in on the form.

Recall that in July of 1815 the Apothecaries' examiners had originally specified *medical* practice, not just any experience observing practitioners in a charity institution. This decision was clearly the only innovation which the examiners introduced into their requirements, for, while hundreds of students attended the hospitals each year, a comparatively small number signed up to follow the staff physicians or apothecaries on their medical rounds. The data available for four of the general hospitals show the thriving state of surgical practice (see Figure 2.2). These hospitals, moreover, certainly had more pupils following the staff surgeons or physicians than those who actually named Guy's, St. Thomas's, St. George's, or the Middlesex on their Apothecaries' registration forms. At St. Thomas's and the Middlesex, for example, of the 61 physicians' pupils between 1815 and 1819, only 33 (54 per cent) applied for an Apothecaries' licence, while 28 (46 per cent) did not.[34] No numerical data are available for the dispensaries, but it is likely that only a handful of young men sought out their physicians for medical experience before 1815.[35]

Faced with the fact that most (five out of eight) of the applicants in August and early September 1815 had surgical, rather than medical, experience in the London hospitals, in late September 1815 the examiners resolved 'That for the present such candidates for examination as shall have attended the practice of an hospital for six months, shall be admitted, provided they shall have otherwise complied with the regulations of the court.'[36] How long this resolution was in force is unclear; in the summer of 1819 the examiners still accepted students with evidence of only surgical practice, although there are no hints that the relaxation of the medical requirement had been publicized.

The printed, formal regulations, in fact, appear to have spurred on the development of medical practice at London

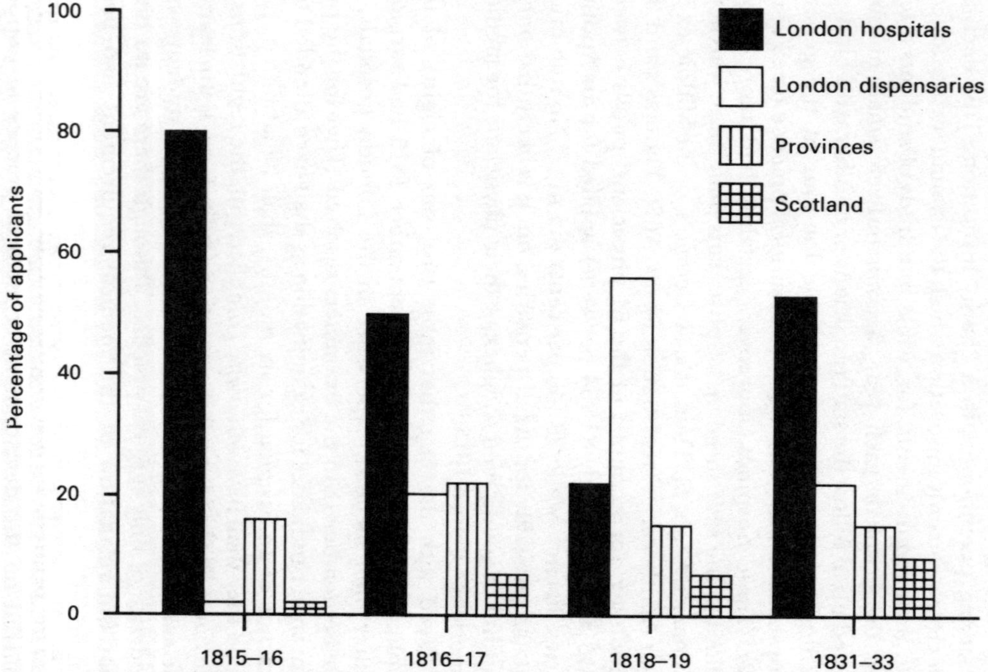

Figure 2.1 Apothecaries' candidates: distribution of clinical practice, 1815–19 and 1831–3

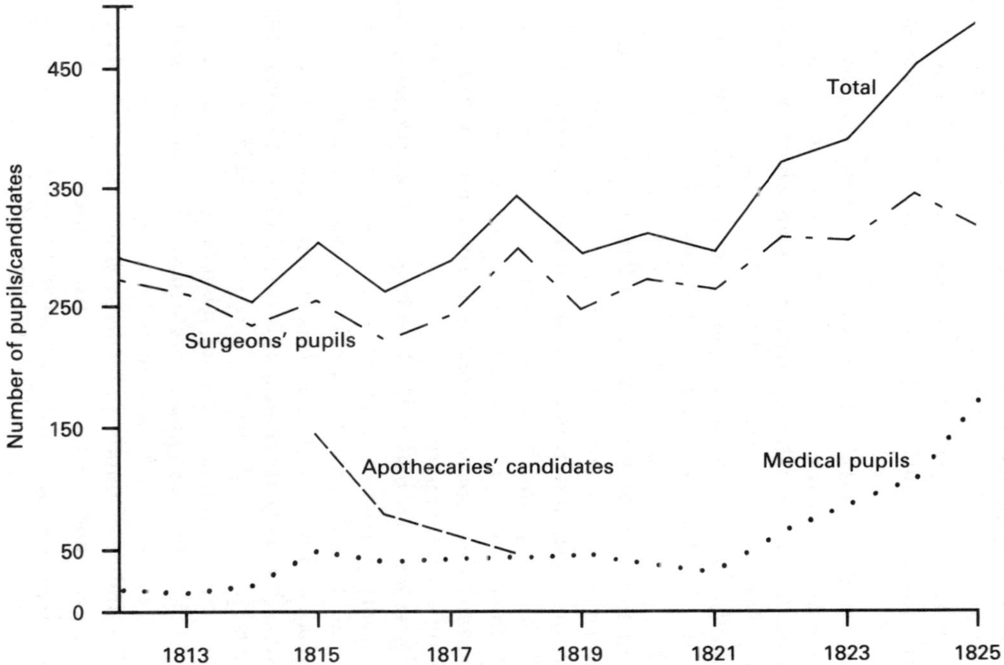

Figure 2.2 London hospital pupils and Apothecaries' licences: Guy's, St. Thomas's, St. George's, and the Middlesex, 1812–25

dispensaries, the most popular of which were the Marylebone, the Surrey, and the General Dispensary on Aldersgate Street. By 1818–19, as Figure 2.1 shows, only 22 per cent of the applicants went to a London hospital, while 56 per cent attended a dispensary or infirmary. London still attracted at least three-quarters of the students, but the distribution had shifted dramatically.

There are several overlapping reasons for this migration. First, dispensaries were somewhat less expensive than the hospitals. The evidence is sparse, but during the late eighteenth century physicians' pupils at the hospitals paid between twenty and twenty-five guineas for a year's attendance. At St. Thomas's before 1815, physicians' pupils could follow the medical practice for six months for fifteen guineas, while Guy's physicians asked only ten guineas for half a year. Also, special rates were available at these two hospitals for surgeons' pupils who wished to attend the medical rounds, although at St. Thomas's that arrangement ended in 1812.[37] It is likely that a similar scale of fees existed at the other general hospitals when the Apothecaries' Act came into effect. Unfortunately, no information is presently available on the comparative costs of dispensary practice. In 1825, however, the *Lancet* published its sweeping review of all opportunities for medical education in London. According to this report, dispensary physicians in London charged between five and seven guineas for six to nine months' attendance; the Westminster, in contrast, was the least expensive hospital, the physicians there asking nine guineas for six months, while the others demanded between ten and twelve.[38]

Second, the dispensaries may well have appealed to students seeking clinical experience which more closely resembled private practice than that in the hospitals. As Loudon has shown, dispensary physicians attended a broader range of diseases, from mild conditions to acute fevers, than those admitted to hospital, and went on home visits as well as consulting at their charities.[39] Finally, it seems that between 1815 and about 1821, hospital physicians themselves were not especially eager to promote medical attendance among nascent general practitioners. The reasons for this apparent reluctance are complex and, at present, obscure. Perhaps some of them preferred instructing a small number of pupils, particularly young men intending to take degrees and become physicians themselves. Some Fellows of the Royal College of Physicians may well have stood on their dignity, intimidating potential students with their demeanour, if not with their medical knowledge, experience, and price. In any case, the London hospitals' staff, with their plethora of surgeons' pupils, initially carried on as though the Apothecaries' Act hardly existed.

In the first years of the Act, therefore, the London dispensary physicians offered medical experience that was probably less expensive, more suited to preparation for general practice, and more congenial than that provided in the London hospitals. By the early 1830s, however, as the data presented to the Select Committee on Medical Education show, the London hospitals had regained their dominance over clinical instruction, attracting at least 53 per cent of the applicants registered between 1831 and 1833.

Precisely how and when the London hospitals moved back into first place is complicated and as yet unclear. The hospitals' ascendancy undoubtedly stemmed from broader changes in medical education in London that the Society of Apothecaries both responded to and encouraged in the late 1820s and 1830s. It is worth stressing, however, that the shift does not correspond simply to the creation of hospital 'schools' where the staff conveniently offered lectures on the hospitals' grounds. The physicians and surgeons at Guy's, St. Thomas's, St. Bartholomew's, and the London had constructed nearly complete schools by the 1790s. These continued, with varying curricula, throughout the years when the dispensaries were popular clinical alternatives. The Middlesex, St. George's, and the Westminster, in contrast, had ward-walking pupils who depended upon nearby extramural lectures until the 1830s and 1840s, when these hospitals belatedly caught up with those who had in-house courses.[40]

The hospitals' ultimate success in capturing the market for medical teaching probably lay partially in their proponents' claims that they were the most important and significant arenas for clinical experience. During the early 1820s, a new generation of hospital physicians emerged, such as Richard Bright (Guy's), Archibald Billing (the London), Peter Mere Latham (the Middlesex, then St. Bartholomew's), and John Elliotson (St. Thomas's, for whom ward teaching and formal clinical lectures were not only more agreeable, but also vital for the emerging conception of clinical medicine linked to the study of morbid anatomy.[41] In part riding on the coat-tails of Parisian clinicians, but also extending the surgeons' (and some physicians') much older enthusiasm for bedside instruction in the London hospitals, such physicians implicitly asserted the hospitals' role as revitalized centres for social, intellectual, and professional authority.[42]

Whether or not the Apothecaries' examiners consciously accepted the hospital's casting as a pre-eminent medical institution, they certainly responded to, and ultimately supported, its star status. Their institutional differentiation began in 1824, when the examiners decided that nine months' medical practice at a dispensary would be equivalent to six months on a hospital ward. In 1828, they defined a hospital as a medical institution with sixty or more beds, thus distinguishing the hospital from a mere infirmary. In 1829, they increased the required number of months of clinical practice to nine in a hospital or twelve in a dispensary. By this time, the examiners were not content to allow institutions to define themselves. A delegation from the Society, for example, visited the Royal Western Hospital in 1829 and their report led the examiners to rule that 'it was not, in its present state, competent to fulfil the intentions of this court in respect to the physicians' practice, as a hospital'.[43] Finally, on 9 September 1830, the examiners produced a thoroughly revised set of standards for their candidates. They demanded either a year at a hospital whose physicians offered clinical lectures or fifteen months at a hospital without clinical lectures or fifteen months at a dispensary 'connected with some medical school recognized by this court'.[44] That over 50 per cent of their applicants in 1813–3 had chosen a London general hospital, most with clinical lectures, reflects the students' acceptance of the importance of hospital rather than dispensary experience or, perhaps, a pragmatic choice of the slightly shorter time to qualification.[45] The Apothecaries' regulations thus confirmed a hierarchy of medical institutions and, while not overtly discounting dispensary practice, awarded precedence to the larger teaching hospitals. The student, they determined, would learn as much in a year on the wards with clinical lectures as he could in fifteen months of traditional instruction, simply observing the practice of dispensary or ward-walking physicians.[46]

At the same time that the examiners separated hospitals from dispensaries, they also confronted the tensions which emerged during the Act's early years. Possibly in response to the perception that students were increasingly taking the minimum number of necessary courses to sit the licensing examination, the Apothecaries gradually added lecture requirements. In 1826, for example, they demanded certificates of two courses in midwifery and the diseases of women and children, although they did not examine candidates in this subject. In 1827, 1828, and more thoroughly in 1830, they specified the order in which pupils should attend lectures and medical practice.[47] A few years earlier, in 1824, the examiners began implicitly to regulate the open, competitive market that had supported their initial expectations about appropriate qualifications. Not too surprisingly, their first efforts zeroed in on the students' own honesty. 'In consequence of information having been received by the court . . . that various means are resorted to for the purpose of evading those salutory regulations laid down by the court for the attendance of students at hospitals and dispensaries in London . . . 'the examiners insisted that pupils register at Apothecaries' Hall before starting their practices.[48] Over the next six years, the Apothecaries refined their bureaucratic supervision of students' work. In 1828, they prepared their own set of printed certificates that an applicant had to use to prove his attendance at lectures and clinical rounds. In 1830, they extended their monitoring of pre-registration work by forcing the candidate to register all of his courses at the Hall when these began. In a new step, moreover, the examiners determined how many lectures should be given in each course and announced that they accepted certificates only from lecturers 'recognized by this court'.[49] By outlining the qualifications and apparatus an instructor must have in order for his course to count for a student's LSA, the Apothecaries explicitly began to close the open market in medical education.

Within fifteen years, therefore, the Court of Examiners had transformed its administration of the Apothecaries' Act from a fairly flexible – even loose – application of a minimum set of standards and examination to a far more rigidly defined curriculum backed up by its power to 'recognize' hospitals, dispensaries, and lecturers. Although the public emphasis still lay on the examination itself, a common target for snide comments, in fact the Apothecaries' power emerged, nearly unrecognized, in its pre-examination requirements.[50] Criticisms of the Act abounded throughout the 1820s and 1830s. Reformers agitated to abolish the demeaning apprenticeship clause, to outlaw unlicensed practitioners, and, more broadly, to institute an examining body that would remove the artificial distinction between medical expertise (the LSA) and basic surgical skills (associated with the MRCS). The goal was still to have the public recognize and certify, via government legislation, the general practitioner's function and status.[51] Yet it is difficult to estimate how much impact public comments had on the Society of Apothecaries' gradual changes in their requirements, for in these years reformers overwhelmingly attacked what they saw as the more crucial issues of irregular practice. The Apothecaries' reluctance to prosecute unlicensed medical men and their adherence to the outmoded tripartite division of the profession consumed medical agitators, not the examiners' routine certification of educated students or the pre-examination criteria they had chosen.[52] In the 1834 SCME testimony, for example, most witnesses happily or grudgingly admitted that the Apothecaries had done an admirable job in licensing medical men, considering the legislation that circumscribed their work.[53] Given the Society's history of inertia and tendency to respond to, rather than to create, innovations in medical education, their changing regulations probably reflected underlying shifts in professional and social expectations about medical qualifications, compounded by their own bureaucratic reaction to students' disingenuous claims and the complexities of dealing with a vast array of private and hospital schools.[54]

In conclusion, an analysis of the Society's registration books between 1815 and 1819 highlights pivotal years in the history of British medical education. The Apothecaries' Act of 1815, through the power it gave the examiners to establish educational criteria, at first generally recognized the standards which many pupils had chosen voluntarily. Private enterprise had created a flourishing educational industry in London, and it seemed that it would serve the public's interest to require that all apothecaries have some of the courses and clinical experience which competing medical men offered so eagerly. The fluidity of the 'open' market is particularly apparent in the dispensaries' early success in attracting pupils to their medical practices.

Having more practitioners take courses and observe clinical techniques may well have benefited the public, but, as the Apothecaries' records indicate, regulation had its own subtle effect on medical qualifications. By the end of the fourth year of the Act, the Society's licences went to men who increasingly filled the minimum requirements yet, as a group, were attending fewer courses and spending fewer months with the sick and dying poor. Faced with qualifications tending towards the middle range, and later concern over the ease with which applicants submitted evidence of work that they did not do, the examiners instituted more complex procedures and, by the late 1820s and early 1830s, longer and more exacting course and practice demands. As schools, hospitals, infirmaries, and dispensaries multiplied throughout England, moreover, the Society of Apothecaries began to certify lecturers and to dictate what defined a hospital suitable for clinical experience. Impersonal rules replaced the examiners' personal knowledge of teachers and institutions; comprehensive requirements replaced previously inadequate minimums. The wide diversity of independent lecturers, small schools, and private theatres gradually disappeared as the 'open' market in medical instruction – and the profession – closed. The Apothecaries' Act, however deficient it was in 1815, pointed directly to the mass monitoring, standardization, and rote testing which characterizes modern medical education.

Notes

1. I am grateful to the Department of History and the Office of Research, Ball State University, for the release time and financial support which enabled me to prepare this essay, and to Andrew Wear, for his constructive comments on an earlier draft. An NEH Travel to Collections Grant also contributed to my research costs.

2. For a recent survey of the range of historical interpretations about the Apothecaries' Act, see Irvine Loudon, *Medical Care and the General Practitioner, 1750–1850* (Oxford, 1986), pp. 129–88. The now standard account of the Act is that of S. W. F. Holloway, 'The Apothecaries' Act, 1815: a reinterpretation', *Medical History*, 10 (1966), 107–29, 221–36, who also reviews the literature praising the Act's influence. Typical of such positive views is that of F.N.L. Poynter, who described the Act as 'a turning point in medical education': 'Medical education in England since 1600', in C.D. O'Malley (ed.), *The History of Medical Education* (Berkeley, 1970), p. 240.

3. Loudon, *Medical Care and the General Practitioner*, pp. 172–3; M. Jeanne Peterson, *The Medical Profession in Mid-Victorian London* (Berkeley, 1978), pp. 22–30; Judy Sadler, 'Ideologies of "art" and "science" in medicine: the transition from medical care to the application of technique in the British medical profession', in W. Krohn, E.T. Layton, Jr, and P. Weingart (eds), *The Dynamics of Science and Technology* (Dordrecht, 1978), pp. 177–93; Ivan Waddington, *The Medical Profession in the Industrial Revolution* (Dublin,

1984). In 'Medical education in England, 1830–1858: a sociological analysis', *History*, 49 (1964), 299–324, S. W. F. Holloway argued that 1830–58 was the crucial period for the formulation of modern medical education, primarily stressing regulations and the formal unification of the profession. I argue, here and elsewhere, that the organization of medical education in England had much longer roots which effectively shaped the regulations ultimately imposed.

4. For reference to these sources, see Loudon, *Medical Care and the General Practitioner*, Holloway, 'The Apothecaries' Act'; Great Britain, Parliamentary Papers, *Report of the Select Committee on Medical Education* (SCME), PP 1834, 602, I, II, and III, and Appendices.

5. Guildhall Library, MS 8241/1, Society of Apothecaries, Court of Examiners, 'Entry books of qualifications of candidates, 1815–1819'. David Van Zwanenberg has used these records for a regional study of medical practitioners in his 'The training and apprenticeship of those apprenticed to apothecaries in Suffolk, 1815–1858', *Medical History*, 27 (1983), 139–50.

6. The argument offered in this essay is, as yet, limited to specific developments surrounding the Apothecaries' Act. Parallel changes within the Royal College of Surgeons, who also acted to increase their regulatory power over applicants for the surgeon's diploma, and the precise relationship between the Act and the growth of London and provincial medical schools throughout the 1820s and 1830s, await further re-evaluation.

7. Loudon, *Medical Care and the General Practitioner*, pp. 11–28, 142–6; Bernice Hamilton, 'The medical professions in the eighteenth century', *Economic History Review*, 2nd ser., 4 (1951), 141–69; Cecil Wall, *A History of the Worshipful Society of Apothecaries, 1617–1815*, ed. E. Ashworth Underwood (London, 1963); Sir George Clark, *A History of the Royal College of Physicians of London*, 3 vols, (London, 1966), II, pp. 163, 507–12.

8. Joan Lane, 'The role of apprenticeship in eighteenth century medical education in England,' in W. F. Bynum and Roy Porter (eds), *William Hunter and the Eighteenth Century Medical World* (Cambridge, 1985), pp. 57–104.

9. These points and the following discussion are based on: Loudon, *Medical Care and the General Practitioner*, pp. 39–53; Roy Porter, 'Medical education in England before the teaching hospital: some recent revisions', in John Wilkes (ed.), *The Professional Teacher: Proceedings of the 1985 Annual Conference of the History of Education Society* (London, 1986), pp. 29–44; Susan Lawrence, 'Entrepreneurs and private enterprise: the development of medical lecturing in London, 1775–1820', *Bulletin of the History of Medicine* (forthcoming, June 1988); Susan Lawrence, 'Science and medicine at the London hospitals: the development of teaching and research, 1780–1815', PhD thesis, University of Toronto, 1985. Lisa Rosner's work on Edinburgh education in the eighteenth century also reveals a significant proportion of young men who attended lectures without intending to receive the MD degree. Like those who came to London, these students voluntarily sought knowledge without the expense of formal

certification. Lisa Rosner, 'Students and apprentices: medical education at Edinburgh University, 1760–1810', PhD thesis, Johns Hopkins University, 1985.

10. Lawrence, 'Entrepreneurs and private enterprise,'; Lawrence, 'Science and medicine at the London hospitals', pp. 659–60. See Figure 2.2.

11. Richard Kay, *The Diary of Richard Kay, 1751–61, of Baldingstone, near Bury: A Lancaster Doctor*, ed. William Brockbank and F. Kenworthy (Manchester, 1968), p. 80; V. Mary Crosse, *A Surgeon in the Early Nineteenth Century* (Edinburgh and London, 1968), pp. 31–57; see also John M. T. Ford (ed.), *A Medical Student at St. Thomas's Hospital, 1801–1802: The Weekes Family Letters, Medical History*, Supplement no. 7 (London, 1987); Lawrence, 'Science and medicine at the London hospitals', chs. 5, 10; Loudon, *Medical Care and the General Practitioner*, pp. 34–53.

12. Loudon, *Medical Care and the General Practitioner*, pp. 166–88.

13. Guildhall Library, MS 8200/10, Society of Apothecaries, Court of Assistants, 'Minute Book, 1806–1817'.

14. George Man Burrows, *A Statement of the Circumstances connected with the Apothecaries' Act and its Administration* (London, 1817), p. 9; Loudon, *Medical Care and the General Practitioner*, p. 169.

15. Burrows, *A Statement of the Circumstances*, pp. 9–13. For an account of the fees each examiner earned by sitting on the Court, see SCME, 601–III, Appendix, No. 16. The examiners' remunerations ranged between £45 and £70 annually during the first four years of the Act. For each candidate approved the Court received three guineas, which was divided among those present at the examination. The Court usually met once a fortnight.

16. See, for example, Thomas Beddoes, *A Letter to the Right Honorable Sir Joseph Banks, Bart., on the causes and removal of the prevailing discontents, imperfections and abuses, in medicine* (London, 1808), p. 81. For a summary of later criticisms, see Loudon, *Medical Care and the General Practitioner*, pp. 176–80.

17. Lawrence, 'Entrepreneurs and private enterprise'.

18. Zachary Cope, 'The influence of free dispensaries upon medical education in Britain', *Medical History*, 13 (1969), 29–32.

19. Hamilton, 'The medical professions', pp. 149–50, 166–7; Zachary Cope, *The Royal College of Surgeons of England: A History* (London, 1959), p. 43. See Royal College of Surgeons of England, Library, 'Minutes and Resolutions of the Royal College of Surgeons' Court of Examiners', I, 26 April 1809, 15 June, 7 December 1810, 4 October 1811, 6 August 1813, for the gradual enunciation of vague course and practice requirements.

20. In all of the reforming literature before 1825, only one radical proposal appeared that suggested that lecturers themselves should be certified to teach. In 1813, the Association of Apothecaries and Surgeon-Apothecaries offered a bill that would include a joint committee 'to appoint persons to teach and to give lectures'. Charles Newman, *The Evolution of Medical Education in the Nineteenth Century* (London, 1957), p. 66.

21. The clerk only rarely stated the reason why an examiner failed a candidate. A separate record of rejections was begun on 30 November 1821. It shows that many marginal students failed the first part of the examination when they were unable to translate Latin prescriptions and passages accurately. Guildhall Library, MS 8249/1, Society of Apothecaries, Court of Examiners, 'Examiners notes on candidates referred, 1820–29'.

22. The clerks also developed certain formulaic entries. While they at first noted the precise age of the candidate, after a few months they simply wrote 'of full age', indicating that the applicant was 21 or over. The records could not be used, therefore, to give an age profile of aspiring apothecaries during the period of this study. The clerk began to record ages again in 1823. See Van Zwanenberg, 'The training and apprenticeship of those apprenticed to apothecaries in Suffolk', p. 141, for a table of the ages at the start of apprenticeship for the subgroup apprenticed in Suffolk 1823–53.

23. Students also intending to become members of the Royal College of Surgeons (MRCS) between 1813 and 1819 were required to have attended courses on anatomy and surgery, plus twelve months' hospital attendance. In February 1819, the RCS regulations were made more precise, specifying that each student should have taken two courses in anatomy, one course in surgery, two courses of dissection, and have completed twelve months' attendance on the surgical practice of a large hospital in London, Edinburgh, Glasgow, or Dublin. See Royal College of Surgeons Library, 'Minutes and Resolutions of the Court of Examiners, 1763–1825', 25 February 1819. How many students took both the LSA and the MRCS remains to be investigated through a cross-check of their manuscript registers. Only two of the Apothecaries' candidates between 1 August 1815 and 31 July 1819 were noted as already members of the RCS.

24. Only one student is, as yet, positively known to have under-represented the extent of his qualifications. John Sharpe, who took his Apothecaries' examination on 8 May 1817, had been apprenticed for seven years and had taken two courses in each of the required subjects. He had followed the physicians' practice for a year at the Warrington Dispensary and submitted evidence of a further six months as a surgeons' pupil at the Middlesex Hospital. The Middlesex pupil registers, however, show that he had signed up for twelve months' practice with the surgeons on 3 October 1817, seven months of which had expired when he appeared at the Hall (Middlesex Hospital Archives, Register of Surgeons' Pupils, 1763–1845). It is likely, considering his record, that he intended to apply for the MRCS as well when he had completed his year at the Middlesex. His under-representation in May of 1817, furthermore, was hardly significant, as Sharpe had already exceeded the Apothecaries' minimum requirements. Further evidence on the degree of 'under-represented' candidates must await a lengthy cross-check of all the surviving pupil registers in London.

25. The examination itself was conducted by one of the twelve members of the Court of Examiners, appointed from members of the

Society of Apothecaries. They tested the student by 1) a translation of prescriptions from Latin and 2) questions 'in the theory and practice of medicine, in pharmaceutical chemistry, and materia medica'. From 1817, they also asked questions on physiology and medical botany (SCME, 601-III, Appendix No. 24; Loudon, *Medical Care and the General Practitioner*, pp. 167–70). Note that the examiners did not question applicants on anatomy, although students were required to complete two courses in the subject.

26. SCME, 602-III, Appendix No. 7. My annual figures disagree slightly with those presented by the Society of Apothecaries in their report. The candidates who first failed and later retook the examination, for example, have two entries in the register. I included them with the cohort of their original application if they later passed with no additional course work or clinical practice, since their technical requirements were completed with the earlier group. The Society's clerk appears to have counted such students twice, first as rejected applicants and then as passes in another year. The difference between the figures is not significant, except for the 1818–19 group whose outcome is not known from the registration forms. A more refined analysis would require that the information from the forms be carefully compared with the brief notes taken on each examination, compiled in Guildhall Library, MS 8239/1, Society of Apothecaries, Court of Examiners, 'Minute Book, 1815–19'.

27. Loudon, *Medical Care and the General Practitioner*, p. 167, notes that the London certificate cost ten guineas, while a country one cost only six guineas. Those transferring from the country to London were required to make up the difference in a special application to the Society.

28. These were, with the dates of their registration forms, Archibald Armstrong (4 April 1816), who had eleven years in the army; William Parker (18 April 1816), with an unspecified term in the 29th Regiment of Foot as surgeon; John Scatehand (25 April 1816), a surgeon in the Royal Navy; and Lemmard Stoaker (30 May 1816), who had served four years with the West Essex Militia.

29. John Bacot, chairman of the Court of Examiners from 1832, was quizzed by the SCME about the apparently low rate of failures in the early years of the Act (an average of 1 in 16.6 for 1815–19, or 6 per cent according to the Society's figures) compared with later ones (1 in 6, or nearly 17 per cent, for 1830–4). Bacot attributed the higher failure rate to the higher educational standards of the later period. John Ridout, an examiner since 1815, thought the rejection rate increased after Celsus and Gregory had been added to the texts which students should be able to translate on sight, although he admitted the problem might also lie with the crowding in clinical practice. Finally, John Watson, secretary to the Court of Examiners in 1834, thought that the shift in failure rates reflected better examiners (SCME, 602-III, pp. 28, 38, 43, 50). The increasing failure rates may also reflect the examiners' loss of flexibility in the face of increasingly specific requirements and concern over the Society's reputation, which obliged them to refer (fail) more applicants. An analysis of the latter registers is necessary to ascertain this point.

30. Burrows, *A Statement of Circumstances*, pp. 16–37, Appendix No. VII, pp. vii–x.

31. Cope, 'The influence of free dispensaries upon medical education in Britain,' pp. 29–36; Mary J. Chamard, 'Medicine and the working class: the dispensary movement in London, 1867–1911', PhD thesis, University of Toronto, 1984, p. 56.

32. Irvine Loudon, 'The origins and growth of the dispensary movement', *Bulletin of the History of Medicine*, 55 (1981), 341, n. 45.

33. The percentages shown in the figure for 1815–19 were calculated from among the candidates who chose only one institution (a London hospital, or dispensary, etc.). Those who followed medical staff at more than one location, a provincial hospital and a London dispensary for example, were omitted from this analysis in order to give clear data of students' preferences. Counting each separate entry for clinical work, moreover, offered similar proportions: in 1815–16, for example, 72 per cent attended a London hospital, 5 per cent a London dispensary, 12 per cent a provincial hospital or dispensary, 4 per cent Edinburgh and Glasgow, and 6 per cent had military experience in practice or at a military hospital.

34. St. Thomas's Hospital Medical School Library, 'Register of physicians' pupils, 1729–1832'; Middlesex Hospital Archives, 'Register of physicians' pupils, 1766–1840'. These figures include all the applicants who registered for the physicians' practice at St. Thomas's or the Middlesex, although a few did not specify this category on their Apothecaries' form.

35. Cope, 'The influence of free dispensaries upon medical education in Britain', pp. 30–2.

36. SCME, 602-III, Appendix, No. 24. The original resolution appears in Guildhall Library, MS 8239/1, Society of Apothecaries, Court of Examiners, 'Minute Book 1815–19', 28 September 1815.

37. Thomas Champney, *Medical and Chirurgical Reform Proposed from a Review of the Healing Art . . . with Considerations on Hospitals, Dispensaries, Poor Houses and Prisons* (London, 1797), pp. 45–9; flyleaf and loose undated sheet in Guy's Hospital Medical School, Secretary's Office, 'Entry of physicians, surgeons pupils and dressers, 1778–1813'; St. Thomas's Hospital Medical School Library, 'Register of physicians' pupils, 1729–1832'. These figures do not include small extra fees paid to register as a pupil. Probably in response to the dispensaries' (and Guy's) competition, the St. Thomas's physicians gradually reduced their fees: in 1818, the St. Thomas's physicians' practice cost twelve guineas for six months; in 1824, the fee had been lowered to eleven guineas.

38. *Lancet* (1825–6) 1 October 1825, 18–32.

39. Loudon, 'The origins and growth of the dispensary movement', pp. 334–8.

40. Lawrence, 'Entrepreneurs and private enterprise'.

41. 'Account of the metropolitan hospitals, medical schools and lectures for the session commencing October 1832', *Lancet* (1832–33), 3–11. Wakley particularly praised Dr Billing's and Dr Latham's clinical teaching in this survey. William Munk (comp.), *Roll of the Royal College*

of Physicians of London, 2nd edn, 3 vols, (London, 1878), III, pp. 155–60, 185–90, 203–4, 258–63. Russell C. Maulitz, *Morbid Bodies: Pathological Anatomy in England and France* (Cambridge, 1987).

42. Lawrence, 'Science and medicine at the London hospitals', chs 8, 12.

43. SCME, 602-III, Appendix, No. 24, 2 July 1829.

44. These regulations were reprinted SCME, 602-III, Appendix, No. 24.

45. In 1831–3, the physicians at the London, St. Thomas's, Guy's, St. George's, and St. Bartholomew's offered clinical lectures along with ward-walking; the Middlesex and the Westminster did not: *Lancet* (1832–33), 3–11; (1833–4), 3–12. The returns given in SCME, 602-III, Appendix, No. 30 show that, for these years, only seventy-five students attended the Middlesex and the Westminster (excluding the handful who submitted certificates from multiple clinical practices), or just 11 per cent of the total (699) who obtained their certificates from only one of these seven hospitals.

46. SCME, 602-III, p. 44.

47. SCME, 602-III, Appendix, No. 24.

48. SCME, 602-III, Appendix, No. 24, 28 Oct. 1824.

49. SCME, 602-III, Appendix, No. 23, 18 Nov. 1830; see also, Society of Apothecaries, *A Statement by the Society of Apothecaries on the Subject of their Administration of the Apothecaries' Act* (London, 1844), Appendix, 'Preface to the Regulations of the Court of Examiners issued in September 1830', pp. 40–4.

50. For belittling reactions to the Apothecaries' examination, see Loudon, *Medical Care and the General Practitioner*, p. 173; 'Opinions of a radical reformer', *Lancet* (1826–7), 455–6.

51. Loudon, *Medical Care and the General Practitioner*, pp. 171–88; Holloway, 'The Apothecaries' Act, 1815: a reinterpretation', pp. 224–32.

52. Holloway, 'The Apothecaries' Act, 1815: a reinterpretation', pp. 233–5.

53. Society of Apothecaries, *A Statement . . . on the Subject of their Administration of the Apothecaries' Act*, pp. 19–24.

54. Society of Apothecaries, *A Statement . . . on the Subject of their Administration of the Apothecaries' Act*, pp. 9, 14. In this 1844 account, the Society summarized its history: '[A]s the means of acquiring professional knowledged increased, the Court have cautiously and gradually increased their demands upon the students, extending their curriculum of study, and raising the standards of examination' (p. 9).

3

'Trading assassins' and the licensing of anatomy

Ruth Richardson

Most readers probably know nothing of the Anatomy Act of 1832. It is an obscure piece of legislation, and there are few reasons why anyone should have come across it, or, having done so, why they should expend any great effort on it. Most standard histories of medicine either ignore it altogether or refer to it only in passing; and, considering how much there is to say about the history of medicine as a whole, it is probably not too surprising that the Anatomy Act should hitherto have received little attention. The Act is no more than a footnote in medical history. Yet I hope to show that it is an important footnote.

Before we go any further, I have a few points to make concerning the researching and writing of medical history which may hearten those so occupied. We are all fallible. All authors make mistakes. The writers of the standard histories of medicine – whom I do not mean to name – may simply not have had time to research every footnote in detail. And it would be both unfair and unrealistic if we as readers and historians were to demand such devotion to duty on their part. Lives are busy. In the compilation of an encyclopaedic work on the history of medicine, it is obvious that one has to concentrate on the most important topics and lean to a sometimes irksome degree on secondary sources. Despite our own ideals and the wishes of reviewers, it simply isn't possible to be right about everything all of the time, least of all about a footnote.

While, on the one hand, poor scholarship is indefensible, the demand for perfection is unrealistic. As scholars we have continually to strive for a decent balance. It helps, I think, to recognize that in historical work *chance* is more important than is generally appreciated or admitted. One can research a subject for weeks and months and even years, and think one knows it pretty well, when later, in an unexpected context, one may find by chance a document or a piece of information which adjusts one's view. Had we not discovered it, we might have gone forward happily believing in our previous knowledge. Views can be changed in important ways simply because evidence sometimes emerges fortuitously from the great soup of historical source material.

This has certainly occurred many times in my own experience and in that of other historians with whom I've discussed historical writing and research on a personal level. Indeed, I am quite willing to believe that I myself may have missed finding a history of medicine which contains all the material I am about to set down in this chapter. I have, of course, looked at all the major and minor works I can find. But if any reader knows of one which deals with the Anatomy Act in the way I do here, I would be more than pleased to hear of it, and to revise my arguments accordingly.[1]

Another point concerns footnotes. Scholarly footnotes have a propensity to take up a lot of space, they disrupt the flow of reading, their small print is often hard to read and their references often difficult to trace. Examples of books, and especially of theses, exist whose footnotes seem to occupy more column inches than does the text, and upon which the editor's pen could have been applied with rigour.

Nevertheless, footnotes can be very interesting things. One can often find in a footnote enough to keep one busy for a long time. And one's findings can be unexpected, new, exciting, and valuable.

The Anatomy Act is a case in point. It is generally considered worthy of a footnote as it was the instrument by which dissection for anatomy was at last put on a secure legal footing in Britain. The Act was passed by Parliament in the summer of 1832, enacting recommendations laid down by a House of Commons Select Committee, whose findings had been published four years earlier, in 1828.

I found out about the Anatomy Act by accident. I was studying Mary Shelley's novel *Frankenstein*, during a course of study on the Gothic novel, and became curious to know if Frankenstein's fictional research on charnel-house corpses was historically related to Burke and Hare and the body-snatchers. The results of my enquiry subsequently developed into my doctoral thesis, and then my book, *Death, Dissection and the Destitute* – to which colleagues now refer as a deep disquisition on dark and dastardly deeds.[2] When it hasn't been ignored or missed, the Anatomy Act has hitherto been the subject of a clutch of misapprehensions. It is my intention in this chapter to try to correct the record.

The first two words of my title, 'trading assassins', are those of Thomas Wakley, founder editor of the *Lancet*.[3] His phrase refers to the shocking series of murders committed by Burke and Hare in Edinburgh in 1828, crimes which in fact serve as a good starting point for a correction of the historical record.

The first misapprehension is that the Anatomy Act was passed as a direct result of the discovery of the Burke and Hare murders. Now this is not strictly true. A chronological account of events reveals the story to be rather more complicated than that.

Before the Anatomy Act was passed in 1832 dissection was a much hated and feared aggravation of the death sentence only in certain cases of murder. Its potency was located in the fact that dissection effectively denied the wrongdoer a grave. Judiciary and people in Britain were agreed that dissection constituted a fate worse than death. Because of shortages of corpses from gallows, by the time the law was changed in 1832 body-snatching had been going on for at least 150 years – plagued by sporadic detection and public disorder. There were riots at gallows when surgeons attempted to take the bodies of criminals for dissection,[4] and violent disturbances erupted in graveyards and at anatomy schools when cases of grave-robbery came to light.[5]

Although many major discoveries and surgical developments were made during the period, it was not an easy time to be an anatomist. During this long period – between the late seventeenth and the early nineteenth century, Government did little other than make *ad hoc* official secret arrangements to protect particular personnel involved in the traffic.[6] Nothing more general was done to aid the anatomists or to prevent public disturbances associated with body-snatching.

By the 1820s a situation had been reached in which some sort of change in the law seemed necessary. The law reformer Jeremy Bentham drafted an early version of the Anatomy Act after a correspondence on the subject with Peel in 1826.[7] Bentham was himself rather preoccupied with anatomy for personal as well as political reasons: he planned to bequeath his own body for dissection and subsequent reassembly in order to create an *'auto-icon'*, or self-image. In fact the object he directed to be produced – his skeleton clothed in his own clothes, and seated in his chair – may be seen in its glass case at University College, London, today.[8] Bentham's draft anatomy bill proposed that those dying in institutions should be given over for dissection: a crucial change which would effectively define poverty rather than crime as the qualification for dissection.

Very little happened for a couple of years after Bentham's draft bill, until case law swiftly altered everything. In February/March 1828, after years in which body-snatchers had borne alone the brunt of prosecutions for body-snatching, two doctors were prosecuted and convicted of illegality associated with body-snatching. The judgment passed down in March 1828 by Baron Hullock, the judge in one of these cases, was of the utmost significance. It stated that, since the only legal source of corpses was the gallows, all other sources were illegal.[9] This crucial judgment rendered all anatomists vulnerable to the charge of criminality they had for so long managed to avoid, and provoked a swift response from Parliament. A House of Commons Select Committee was set up within forty days. The committee took evidence during April and May 1828, and its report was then written up and published in July 1828, immediately before the summer recess. The *Report* endorsed Bentham's recommendations.[10]

It was not until Hallowe'en that year that Burke and Hare committed the last of their sixteen murders. They were detected the following morning – on 1 November 1828 – and their victim's corpse was retrieved from Dr Knox's dissection rooms. The advent of 'burking' had at last provided proof positive that market forces operating in the supply of corpses for dissection resulted in multiple murder.

The first Anatomy Bill was submitted to Parliament on 12 March 1829, amid a wave of national revulsion against the murders, but it was withdrawn on 5 June 1829 on the advice of the Duke of Wellington. The run up to what was to become the Reform Crisis was under way by this time, and the Duke probably feared that the Bill would be contentious and might perhaps provoke trouble.

There the matter rested for two-and-a-half-years, until a new case of murder for anatomy was detected in London. Bishop and Williams, who became known as the 'London Burkers', were discovered on 5 November 1831, almost precisely three years after Burke and Hare. Bishop and Williams confessed only to the murder of three poor street folk, but they were widely believed to have dispatched at least sixty people to their deaths. The furore surrounding this second case of burking was the cue for the submission of a new Anatomy Bill to Parliament – on 15 December 1831, only ten days after Bishop and Williams had been hanged and dissected. This second bill passed through Parliament swiftly, in the wake of the Great Reform Bill, and received the Royal Assent on 1 August 1832.

From this chronology, it would seem fairly clear that, although there does exist a relationship between Burke and Hare and the Anatomy Act, this relationship is not the simple one generally proposed. The Act which passed through Parliament in 1832 was composed along broadly similar lines to the bill laid out by Bentham in 1826. Both Bentham and the parliamentary Select Committee had recommended the changes subsequently enshrined in law before Burke and Hare had ever been heard of. Although the first bill's parliamentary progress was undoubtedly affected by Burke and Hare, Parliament's reaction to their crimes was not sufficient in itself to ensure the first bill's passage through the Lords. The Act finally reached the statute book after the efforts of two other less well-known criminals provided the occasion for further parliamentary action on the matter. The fact that both Bentham's draft anatomy bill and the publication of the Select Committee recommendations *predated* the discovery of burking would suggest that the effect of burking on the Anatomy Act was contributory, rather than causative. Even had burking never occurred, legislative change was in gestation, along the very lines which later became law.

The notion that Burke and Hare were responsible for the Anatomy Act actually comes, like many other simple and persuasive ideas, from the pen of Thomas Wakley, writing in his journal, the *Lancet*, in 1829.

> Burke & Hare . . . it is said are the real authors of the measure, and that which would never have been sanctioned by the deliberate wisdom of Parliament, is about to be extorted from its fears. . . . It would have been well if this fear had been manifested and acted upon before sixteen human beings had fallen victims to the supineness

> of the Government & Legislature. It required no extraordinary sagacity to foresee, that the worst consequences must inevitably result from the system of traffic between resurrectionists and anatomists, which the executive government has so long suffered to exist. Government is already in a great degree, responsible for the crime which it has fostered by its negligence, and even encouraged by a system of forbearance.[11]

Two important things are noteworthy about this passage: Wakley was in fact arguing his point in the context of the *first* Anatomy Bill, which subsequently failed in the Lords; and he was making a political rather than a historical point.

The **second** misapprehension about the Anatomy Act is related to the first, in that it involves the belief that the Act was passed as a humanitarian measure to prevent further burking, and to assist medicine. I do not seek to sow doubt that assistance to medicine and, later, the prevention of burking were components in the Act's framing and passage, but rather to suggest that other, perhaps more important reasons for the Act's passage have so far been overlooked. The chronology outlined above suggests that differentiation must be made between influential events and strategies by which the Act finally gained its passage and the aims and intentions of those promoting it.

We have seen that what precipitated the appointment of the Select Committee was the successful conviction of two doctors in 1828. The Committee's function was not to prevent burking, which had not then been discovered, but rather to endorse Bentham's project by the adoption of a formula which would not only decriminalize dissection, but would also initiate the contentious project of dissecting the 'unclaimed' poor from hospitals and workhouses.

This conjoint project, one part protective of medicine, the other a shocking aggravation of the humiliation of a death in poverty, was of a piece with contemporary Benthamite ideas. Space precludes detail here, but the Select Committee on Anatomy conforms absolutely with the findings of historians Samuel Finer and Lucy Brown concerning the ways in which parliamentary and government structures were manipulated by Benthamites for their own ends.[12] This in itself is important, for a **third** misapprehension about the Anatomy Act has really been a failure of perception, and it concerns the importance of the

Anatomy Act beyond the medical field: an importance which, again, has been hither to missed.

The Act was in fact very significant on a number of non-medical fronts. Most crucially, the Anatomy Act established the first centrally funded inspectorate of the nineteenth-century Benthamite calendar of government reform. Only one other historian, as far as I can discover, has so far noticed this important event, and not in a standard medical history of medicine.[13] The establishment of the Anatomy Inspectorate set an important precedent for government intervention in the operations of *laissez faire* in other fields. The establishment of an inspectorate was obtained from Parliament in the case of anatomy when it became clear that unfettered trade in corpses was no longer acceptable to the public or the profession. The worsening political situation in the run up to the Great Reform Bill, in which it no longer seemed impossible to select those for dissection on grounds of poverty alone, crucially assisted the establishment of a parliamentary precedent. Within the next decade inspecting departments were established in such fields of concern as factories, lunacy, emigration, poor law, prisons, tithes, education, railways, and mines.[14]

As we have seen, until 1832, dissection had been reserved by law only for murderers. In fact, Burke, Bishop, and Williams were hanged and publicly dissected – the poetic justice of the latter punishment being viewed as peculiarly appropriate for such miscreants. Yet within months of the London burkers' dissection, the Anatomy Act enacted that the same dire punishment should fall instead on those too poor to pay for their own funeral. Henceforth anyone dying in need of a parish burial could legally be requisitioned for dissection.

Those with an understanding of the poverty of the 1830s cannot fail to be aware of what this change must have meant to the poor, and cannot fail to appreciate what contribution the Anatomy Act was to make to the success of the New Poor Law, which was intended to render poor relief so humiliating and painful that poor people would cease to apply for it. In the popular mind, the dissection of the dead came to be identified with the other meannesses and degradations of the New Poor Law – the separation of husbands from wives, and both from their children, their incarceration in the new workhouses, the vilification of unmarried mothers, the provision of minimum subsistence, and the coldness and humiliation so well portrayed in *Oliver*

Twist.[15] At the time the Anatomy Act was proposed, news of its provisions provoked terror among workhouse inmates.[16]

High workhouse mortality of course assisted the implementation of the Anatomy Act, and dissection served to promote the stigma of the pauper's funeral, which as we shall see, served to promote thrift among the poor. They are wise politicians who appreciate the power of a good stigma.

A **fourth** misapprehension about the Anatomy Act is that there existed no alternative to the requisition of the 'unclaimed'. In fact, a great many possible alternatives were proposed at the time.[17] Among the most frequent suggestions were that suicides, duellists, horse thieves, and all criminals dying in prison should be requisitioned rather than the poor. Other ideas put forward at the time included various ways in which the stigma attached to dissection could be allayed and ultimately removed, among them the idea that the King should set a fashion by bequeathing his body for dissection, rather than the customary extensive embalmment, and hence promote the willing donation of corpses from his subjects in all walks of society.

Another scheme was suggested in which the Royal College of Surgeons would administer a scheme whereby a register would be made of future donors, who would be paid a lump sum in their lifetime for bequeathing their body after death. The most exciting of the schemes put forward at the time was one in which the Government would rescind death duties for those who were kind enough to bequeath their own bodies for anatomy. Each of the more feasible schemes embodied the notion that it was the responsibility of Government to do something to promote the development of a modern system of bequest.

None of these alternatives was considered either by the Select Committee or by Parliament. Their feasibility was simply never assessed. This omission in itself supports my suggestion that the proposal to dissect the poor was primarily a political one.

Misapprehension number **five** appears only implicitly in the standard medical histories, but has often been raised by audiences at my lectures, who suppose the Anatomy Act represented a triumph of secularism. The argument goes that to promote and pass such a law the Act's supporters must surely have jettisoned old-fashioned notions of the sanctity of the body. That this reading of the Act is a mistaken one can be demonstrated without difficulty. Before the Anatomy Act, body-snatchers obtained their corpses for sale to the anatomists from fresh graves and vaults. The poor were their primary targets because pit burials offered less resistance to their shovels: cheap coffins were flimsy, and several fresh corpses could be obtained after one spate of digging. Nevertheless, the nature of the business was such that others were also vulnerable: all fresh corpses, whether in graves or vaults, were fair game. The wealthy certainly feared dissection enough to invest in stout coffins, patent iron coffins, cages called 'mortsafes', and other costly expedients to thwart the grave-robbers. Even so, the eminent surgeon-anatomist Sir Astley Cooper was able to say in evidence to the Select Committee that 'there is no person, let his situation in life be what it may, whom, if I were disposed to dissect, I could not obtain'.[18] All social classes were vulnerable.

Under the Anatomy Act, the social derivation of corpses for anatomy was instead restricted to the poorest inmates of hospitals and workhouses. By its provision of this cheap and legal source, the Act was the means whereby the financially fortunate protected their own remains from the predations of the body-snatchers. As one of the Act's critics put it, 'It is a point not to be lost sight of, that all classes of the community had their share of the annoyance [of body-snatching]; all were liable to be reached by it. By the Bill of 1832, the upper and middle classes were protected, while the poor alone were left exposed.'[19]

Such a change hardly represents a triumph of secularism. It serves rather to indicate the strength of the repugnance towards dissection and concern about the repose of their own remains among many of those who promoted the Act. Sir Astley Cooper, whose evidence in support was just quoted, offers a perfect illustration of my point. A brilliant anatomist and surgeon, President of the Royal College of Surgeons, created baronet as a result of his labours as Surgeon to the King, Cooper must have purchased hundreds – if not thousands – of corpses from body-snatchers during the course of his teaching and surgical career. It is said he had such a passion for dissection that he felt unsatisfied if he did not do some dissecting every day, including weekends. Cooper was the first witness to appear before the Select Committee, and strongly supported the expedient of dissecting the workhouse poor. From the considerable size of his own stone sarcophagus, however, which contains at least two, and possibly three inner coffins, it is evident that Cooper meant to ensure that he would not undergo the same fate.[20]

The sixth misapprehension I want to address concerns the Act's specification of the 'unclaimed' as liable for requisition. Under the Act, dissection was confined to those who died alone in an institution – hospital or workhouse – without kin to claim the body. A petition from the Paisley Reform Society against the dissection of the poor argued that 'to talk of the absence of relatives of the pauper as a reason why his remains should not be respected, is to insult the humanity of a Nation professing a creed which teaches that all men are brothers.'[21] The Committee's *Report* dealt with this moral objection by the insertion of a clause which permitted inmates of institutions to make a written declaration before two witnesses to the effect that they didn't want to be dissected.[22]

The clause is a very important one, as it provides a legal precedent for the proposed change in the law to requisition kidneys today. This proposal has so far foundered, as there exists a general recognition that there is an ethical difference between a system of requisitioning all kidneys which allows individuals to opt out, and an opting-in system in which every kidney is a positive gift. Requisition would, of course, yield many more kidneys, but would seed public disquiet.

As the Earl of Eldon pointed out in Parliament, none without consent is very different from all without dissent.[23] The important Anatomy Act clause concerned the requisition of the whole body, yet, although the pauper was offered an opportunity to opt out, there was nothing in the text to ensure that these wishes would be recorded and observed. Moreover, no penalty was specified in cases where a workhouse inmate's wishes were disregarded. Importantly, there was nothing to ensure the registration of the wishes of those who were illiterate. The existence of the clause was not widely known, and since a workhouse inmate registering a wish to be buried whole would have only other inmates – equally powerless – as witnesses, the clause was virtually a mandate for ignoring the wishes of the poor altogether.

Thomas Wakley had argued in the *Lancet* for the enactment of a penalty for ignoring a person's refusal to allow his or her body to be used for dissection. Had such a clause been inserted in the Act, the first inspector appointed under the Anatomy Act could rightfully have been indicted on these very grounds. Surviving Home Office papers reveal that in the only known cases in which attempts were made to register workhouse inmates' wishes concerning the fate of their own corpses after death, the inspector actively attempted to suppress this registration, and even enlisted the assistance of the Poor Law Commissioners to prevent the circulation of information in workhouses.[24] There is little doubt that, had the Act featured an opting-*in* system, or had paupers' wishes to opt *out* been routinely recorded and observed, the Anatomy Act would have failed miserably from the outset.

The Act also purported to respect the feelings of survivors by permitting the 'claiming' of corpses by 'nearest known relatives'. But no secure definition of the verb 'to claim' was ever adopted in committee, during parliamentary debates, or in the wording of the Act itself. To the Act's supporters, the meaning of 'claim' seems to have been either a non-problem or one which was better left unelaborated. The fundamental problem they wished to avoid confronting was that there existed a gulf of difference between a 'claim' by relatives which involved attendance at a parish funeral and that which would involve shouldering the entire costs of a private interment. Despite evidence that families often failed to claim through poverty, the Select Committee chose in their *Report* to attribute it to 'indifference', and used this supposed indifference to argue that no one's feelings would be hurt by the requisition of the dead. It is worth bearing in mind, too, that under the Anatomy Act 'claiming' had to occur within forty-eight hours of death, but the Act failed to specify whether or when relatives were to be informed.[25]

An understanding of how the Act's failure to define 'claiming' adversely affected the poor may be gained from an 1841 case in which Rosanna Rox called upon the Mayor of Newcastle to help her obtain her mother's body from the local surgeons' hall, after it had been forcibly taken from the parish funeral by a gang of men. The body was found immersed in near-boiling water in preparation for flaying – which would have removed all traces of identity. The anatomists' justification for the men's force and the deceit used to obtain the body was that, despite the presence of several grieving mourners, they had taken the corpse for unclaimed, as there were no relatives present. Rosanna Rox had denied kinship through inability to defray the costs of the funeral.[26]

Another case in point is that of Polly Chapman, which was reported in the *True Sun* in December 1832:

> On Monday evening an inquest was held on Mary Ann Chapman, otherwise 'handsome Poll', aged about twenty-two, an unfortunate prostitute, who drowned herself on Wednesday night in a fit of mental derangement in the London Dock. It appeared that the deceased, who had described herself to her unfortunate associates as related to a coach proprietor named Chaplin at Rochester, was of sober and harmless disposition. Through inability to pay her rent she had been turned out of her lodgings on the morning of her suicide. A verdict of 'mental derangement' was returned; and Mr Holiday, the Churchwarden, asked Mr Baker the Coroner, if he could legally give up the body to the London Hospital, as it was not claimed by any relatives. Mr Baker strongly advised him to do so, as an example to prevent suicide amongst unfortunate women.
>
> Several of the latter class of females, who had conducted themselves with great decorum during the proceedings, here begged with tears and the greatest earnestness, to be allowed to pay a mark of respect to their unfortunate companion, by burying her in consecrated ground, for which purpose they had already raised £3 by subscription, and given to an undertaker. They described her as of the best and most inoffensive disposition, and incapable of injuring anyone.
>
> The Coroner, however, replied that it was necessary to make an example. The spirit of the Anatomy Bill would not be acted up to if the body was not given up. Any resurrectionist might claim the body as a friend, and afterwards sell it. A Juror said he thought the London Hospital had bodies enough from the poor-houses; and that the poor creatures present had shewn much good feeling, and ought to have the corpse. Mr Wilson, the Overseer, wished to take the sense of the Jury on the subject. After such discussion it was decided that the body should be sent to the hospital. The announcement of this decision was received with the most bitter lamentations by the females, who appeared much attached to the deceased.[27]

Polly Chapman's inquest throws up several key points. The 'spirit' of the Act, which confined 'claiming' to nearest known relatives, was grasped and promulgated even though the women attending the inquest were bona fide claimants in any ordinary sense. Polly Chapman was not 'unclaimed'. The Anatomy Act alone made her so.

Surviving records of those were in fact requisi- tioned for dissection under the Act reveal that poor people's bodies were taken against their own living will and against the will of their bereaved survivors.

A **seventh** misapprehension is that after the Anatomy Act dissection was no longer a punishment in British law. The Act's supporters had argued that horror of dissection would disappear when it ceased to serve as a punishment for murder. The Polly Chapman case reveals a mutual understanding of coroner, jury and claimants that dissection did in fact remain a punishment of great potency. The coroner's own choice of language highlights the exemplary and deterrent value of dissection, much as does the women's attempt to deflect the punishment by their stress upon Polly's inoffensive and harmless nature. The Anatomy Act merely transferred what had since Tudor times been a punishment for murder to poverty.

A further misapprehension is that the Anatomy Act was a complete success. The Act did render the poor wary of the workhouse and fearful of a pauper's burial, so it succeeded in terms of adding deterrent value to the New Poor Law workhouses. But, in a medical context, the Act was not an unqualified success. Dissecting the poor proved not to be the hoped-for panacea the anatomists had been encouraged to expect. In numerical terms, the Anatomy Inspector did only about as well as the body-snatchers had done before the Act, and only for the first few years of its operation.[28] This was enough to break the profession's dependence on the body-snatchers, as arrangements were made henceforth directly between anatomists and workhouse personnel, effectively eliminating the body-snatcher from the transaction.[29] Within a comparatively short period, the body-snatchers were rendered virtually redundant. After the first few years, however, numbers of corpses obtained under the Act declined, and opposition to and evasion of dissection by various means resulted in severe shortages of legal corpses for dissection, which continued throughout the nineteenth century and well into the twentieth.[30]

This had several unlooked-for results. Although much less common than before, body-snatching continued sporadically throughout the century, especially outside the metropolitan area.[31] Nor could the Act prevent illegal arrangements between workhouse personnel and anatomists or between hospital surgeons and their own mortuary attendants.[32] In the long term, corpse shortage led to the adaptation of teaching methods: anatomists began to turn their minds to corpse conservation and developed a greater appreciation of preservatives. Dissection manuals began to offer more operations per corpse, more students were taught per body, and there was a revaluation of the tuition of pathology by post-mortem in addition to straightforward dissection.[33]

Nor did the Act serve to dampen the competition between rival anatomy schools. All early nineteenth-century anatomy schools were run on a profit basis, and the Anatomy Inspector endeavoured unsuccessfully to institute some sort of fair distribution system – allocating the available bodies by the number of students at any one establishment. He met constant subversion and non-co-operation, especially from the proprietors of schools attached to teaching hospitals, who could always obtain bodies illegally from their own mortuaries, and who objected to donating them to a general distribution system which would benefit their competitors.

Indeed, the Act really marked the beginning of a new phase in a major struggle, particularly in the London area, between the anatomy schools operating within hospitals and those unattached entrepreneurial schools outside, a struggle which was eventually won by the hospital schools. Their ability to requisition direct from their own mortuaries was supplemented by deals struck with parish authorities, who would receive beds for their sick in return for the bodies of their dead. The Inspector of Anatomy was powerless to enforce a fair distribution system, and the Act contributed instead to the demise of the unattached anatomy schools.[34]

Misapprehension number nine is that the Act contributed to the reform of the medical establishment so necessary at the time. In fact, as we have seen, it benefited the hospital/College hierarchy. Moreover, the inspector's power to license anatomy was actually used to maintain exclusivity as between medical professions. For, although physicians and surgeons were permitted licences to dissect and to obtain bodies under the Act, apothecaries were not. Student apothecaries were obliged to study anatomy, but, if they did so by dissection, it had to be under licensed personnel. Apothecaries applying for licences were in fact refused them. Parish doctors were invariably apothecaries, and throughout the nineteenth century, rather than consult better-qualified doctors, the poor used apothecaries much more frequently because their fees were lower. The Act in fact served to reinforce the old demarcations between apothecaries and other medical professionals, which before its passage were beginning to be challenged.[35]

The last misapprehension about the Anatomy Act to be discussed here is the belief that there was no effective opposition to it. In fact, there was very active opposition both within and outside Parliament. The most vocal parliamentary opposition was mounted by 'Orator' Henry Hunt, who tabled amendments to every clause in the entire text; in addition, many petitions were submitted to both Houses against the Act's recommendations.[36] Extra-parliamentary opposition was expressed in terms of riots and even demolitions of anatomy schools during the Act's passage through Parliament.[37] Political and medical opposition to the Act was exemplified by Thomas Wakley – both in his writings in the *Lancet* and in his many speeches at political meetings.[38] Contemporary opponents were quite aware of the political issues involved in the Act, and criticized it on grounds of its infringement of human rights.[39]

Opposition diversified after the Act's passage. Overt opposition continued, particularly in areas of the Midlands and North West where the Anti-Poor Law Movement was strong. Dissenting Guardians of the Poor, who were unwilling to adopt the New Poor Law, were also unwilling to enforce the Anatomy Act. In London, the inspector was driven to enlist the assistance of the Poor Law Commissioners to prevent the circulation in workhouses of anti-Anatomy Act literature informing pauper inmates of their legal rights to a decent burial.[40]

The poor adopted various techniques for avoiding dissection, such as delaying tactics, whereby Victorian sanitary inspectors began to be called to remove bodies kept for days in overcrowded housing. In the 1860s–70s there was an increase in demands for inquests on workhouse inmates. An inquest caused delay, and often involved a post-mortem, both of which would render a corpse unsuitable for dissection.[41]

The most effective way in which the poor avoided death on the parish was by means of insurances and other methods of raising money for funerals. A decade after the Act's passage, Edwin Chadwick commented with some incomprehension that money could be raised from the poor for death insurance when it couldn't be raised for any other purpose – such as health insurance or the education of children.[42] Thrift for death was forced on the British working classes; the alternative was too hideous to contemplate. The importance of death insurance and the stigma of the pauper funeral survived right through the nineteenth century and into our own. In the years just before the Great War, a survey was undertaken by the Fabian Women's Group which revealed that working women with families surviving on about one pound sterling a week regularly spent between 5 and 10 per cent of their pitifully meagre incomes on death insurance.[43] Fears of disposal as a pauper afflict the elderly even today.[44]

So, to sum up, the Anatomy Act has hitherto been subject to a clutch of misapprehensions which it has been the purpose of this chapter to dispel. Though burking doubtless assisted the parliamentary passage of the Anatomy Act, the discovery of Burke and Hare was not in itself sufficient to cause its passage. The Anatomy Act was as much a political as a medical measure. By establishing the first Benthamite Inspectorate, it established a highly important precedent. Moreover, it served to augment the deterrent power of the New Poor Law workhouses. Feasible alternatives to the requisition of the poor were suggested at the time, many of them prefiguring the method of procurement successfully used today. The Act did not represent a triumph of secularism – it merely enabled the financially fortunate to protect their own remains more effectively. The Duke of Wellington, incidentally, was buried in *four* coffins.[45] Poor people were taken for dissection under the Act against their own living will and against the wishes of grieving relatives and friends. The Act was by no means an unqualified success: it provided no more corpses than the body-snatchers had obtained by stealth, it didn't fully put a stop to body-snatching, and it encouraged corruption. The Act sharpened competition between medical schools and contributed to the demise of independent anatomy tuition outside the teaching hospitals. In addition, the Act worked against the reform of the medical professions by disqualifying apothecaries from undertaking dissections. Finally, there was tremendous opposition to the Act, which was evaded and opposed throughout the nineteenth and early twentieth centuries.

Notes

1. I would be glad to hear of any errors or omissions in this chapter. Please write to me at the Institute of Historical Research, University of London, Senate House, Malet Street, London WC1E 7HU.

2. R. Richardson, *Death, Dissection and the Destitute* (Harmondsworth, 1989).

3. *Lancet*, 10 January 1829, 465–6.

4. P. Linebaugh, 'The Tyburn Riot against the surgeons', in D. Hay *et al.*, *Albion's Fatal Tree* (Harmondsworth, 1977).

5. R. Richardson, *Death, Dissection and the Destitute*, pp. 78, 84, 88, 223–6, 228.

6. Ibid., p. 119.

7. R. Richardson, 'Bentham and "bodies for dissection"', *Bentham Newsletter*, 10 (June 1986), 22–33.

8. R. Richardson and B. S. Hurwitz, 'Jeremy Bentham's self-image: an exemplary bequest for dissection', *British Medical Journal*, 295 (18 July 1987), 195–8.

9. *Rex* v. *Davies et al* (1928), Lancaster Assizes, 14 March 1828.

10. R. Richardson, *Death, Dissection and the Destitute*, pp. 107, 331.

11. *Lancet*, 23 March 1829, 818–21.

12. L. Brown, *The Board of Trade and the Free Trade Movement* (Oxford, 1958): S. Finer 'Transmission of Benthamite ideas', in G. Sutherland (ed.), *Studies in the Growth of Nineteenth Century Government* (London, 1972).

13. P. W. J. Bartrip, 'British Government Inspection, 1832–75', *Historical Journal*, 25 (1982), 605–26.

14. Ibid., p. 607.

15. R. Richardson, *Death, Dissection and the Destitute*, pp. 267–70, 358.

16. Ibid., pp. 121–5, 128, 176–9, 221–2, 247, 252, 281, 342, 358.

17. Ibid., ch. 7, 'Alternative necrology', *passim.*

18. Sir Astley Cooper, Evidence to Select Committee on Anatomy (1828), Reply to Question 50.

19. W. Roberts, *Mr Warburton's Anatomy Bill* (London, 1843), p. 8.

20. Sir Astley Cooper's stone sarcophagus may be found in the vaults of Guy's Hospital Chapel, London. His passion for dissection is the liftmotiv of Bransby Cooper's *Life of Sir Astley Cooper* (London, 1843).

21. Petition of the Paisley Reform Society, House of Commons, *Votes & Proceedings*, Appendix (3 February 1832).

22. 2 & 3 Gul. IV, c.75, *An Act for Regulating Schools of Anatomy* (1832).

23. *Hansard*, 2 February 1832, p. 1151.

24. *Lancet*, 11 December 1831, 593. I have to thank Dr Betty Bostetter, Wakley's biographer, for this reference. MH74/12, Public Records Office, London; HO83/1; *Anatomy Inspector's Quarterly Report* (January 1841), Public Records Office, London.

25. *Report of the Select Committee on Anatomy* (1828), pp. 9–10.

26. *Lancet*, 13 March 1841, 876–9. MH74/13; HO83/1, Public Records Office, London.

27. *True Sun* (1 December 1832).

28. R. Richardson, *Death, Dissection and the Destitute*, pp. 245, 290. MH74/16, Public Records Office, London.

29. R. Richardson, *Death, Dissection and the Destitute*, p. 237.

30. Ibid., pp. 235–7, 243–6, 256, 290.

31. Ibid., pp. 237, 245, 263.

32. Ibid., pp. 233–8. The author of a forthcoming biography of the Victorian surgeon Treves, Stephen Trombley, informs me that Treves obtained literally hundreds of bodies in this way.

33. R. Richardson (1988), *op. cit.*, pp. 179, 345.

34. Ibid., p. 249.

35. Ibid., pp. 213–14.

36. Ibid., pp. 175–9, 183–4, 187–9, 199, 202, 204, 221, 224, 292, 343, 347, 367, 373.

37. Ibid., pp. 87, 90–3, 104, 202, 223–6, 228, 264, 325, 372.

38. Ibid., pp. 154–7.

39. See note 36 above.

40. HO83/1; MH74/13; *Anatomy Inspector's Quarterly Report* (January 1841). Public Records Office, London.

41. R. Richardson (1988), *op. cit.*, pp. 278–9. The habits of the Victorian working class in keeping bodies for long periods have always been greeted with horror and incomprehension. I hope that my work will aid understanding.

42. *Report of the Select Committee on the Improvement of Health in Towns: Supplement* (1843), p. 54 [by E. Chadwick].

43. M. P. Reeves, *Round About a Pound a Week* (London, [1913], 1979), pp. 69, 82–7.

44. R. Richardson, *Death, Dissection and Destitute*, p. 280; R. Richardson, 'Death in the metropolis', MA thesis, University of Sussex, 1978.

45. J. Morley, *Death, Heaven and the Victorians* (London, 1971), p. 81.

4

The disappearance of the patient's narrative and the invention of hospital medicine

Mary E. Fissell

In June 1744, the Bristol surgeon Alexander Morgan went to see a man who felt giddy and had pains in his head. Morgan noted down how his patient had fallen ill in the following words,

> The third Day after the Wether happened to be very warm he changed his Thick Waistcot for a Linning one & being careless sat a quarter day in a Room that was wett the same evening he found himself not well & a little Feverish & thirsty for which he Went to Bed & Drank Plentifull of Sack Whey. The Next Morning he was very horse and out of order . . .[1]

While these are Morgan's words, they are also those of his patient. For it was the patient who supplied him with the details of how he came to fall ill and ultimately require Morgan's services. It was the patient who constructed a narrative from the physical manifestations of his or her illness.

Such narratives of illness were the medium of exchange between early modern patients and doctors – be they physicians, surgeons, or apothecaries. Not only did they place doctor and client on near-equal hermeneutic footing, they also provided non-medical men and women with a distinctive framework for understanding episodes of illness. If, as Nicholas Jewson has argued, early modern medicine was dominated by the client, these tales of sickness should reveal the complex negotiations between patient and practitioner that characterized therapeutic relationships.[2] Jewson's model is based upon that of aristocratic clientage, predicated upon élite patients and eager-to-please doctors. But, in modified form, it can explicate doctors' relationships with their more humble clients as well. In particular, Jewson suggests that the lush profusion of eighteenth-century medical theories derived from physicians' needs to differentiate themselves in a crowded market. But on a more plebeian level, medical knowledge was a part of popular culture; patients had a wealth of concepts and remedies upon which to draw. Doctors, I would suggest, lacked control over the production or consumption of such knowledge, and had to tailor their diagnoses and treatment accordingly. Hence, just as Cecil Helman has shown in an analysis of a twentieth-century medical practice, diagnosis and therapeutics were negotiated between doctor and patient.[3]

However, by the middle of the eighteenth century, this common ground was beginning to erode. The relationship between lower-class patients and their doctors was decisively changed within the hospital, and medical knowledge came to mirror this new arrangement. Hospitals of one sort or another had, of course, existed from the Middle Ages. But the provincial voluntary hospital (and some of its metropolitan counterparts) were an eighteenth-century invention.[4] The Bristol Infirmary was founded in 1737 as a charity designed to pull the working man back from the brink of pauperism, to return a sick man or woman to physical health and economic independence.[5] Hospital patients needed letters of recommendation for admission; like other charities, the infirmary was an expression of personal benevolence. However, by the latter half of the eighteenth century, doctors assumed increasing control of the hospital, and the highly personalized nature of its charity slowly evaporated.

It was in this context of increasing medical autonomy that the patient's narrative of illness was made utterly redundant. Hospital medicine came to focus on signs and symptoms, which provided doctors with a disease-orientated diagnosis conducive to the demands of hospital practice and reflective of its social structure. Of course, the patient's narrative did not disappear quickly or completely, even in the hospital. But its erosion was well under way by the turn of the century.

Earlier on, as a patient recounted how he or she fell ill, the story itself was the object of scrutiny by doctor and patient alike. Both were, in effect, able to hold the narrative up to the light and make of it what they would. In Morgan's case, sometimes roles were reversed; he learned from a woman how she had cured herself of lifelong deafness,

> when she was warm at night in her bed she wold stop her mouth and nose very close and indevored to blow her breath as forseable as she could through her nose which in a Little time brought her to her hearing.[6]

Most of the notebook which records Morgan's interactions with his patients seems to have been kept while Morgan was an apprentice; there are numerous references to his master sending him out to see (and to treat) patients. He seems to have used his notebook as a reference work; he indexed it and added to it occasionally over the years. Thus, his careful recording of this woman's cure for deafness put it on an equal plane with his own remedies. Morgan and his patients both were capable of interpreting illness, and Morgan was not necessarily granted the final word.

This interpretative equality implied that both meaning and treatment could be negotiated. For example, a man came to Morgan with an ulcer on his penis. 'I supposed it to be veneriall but by no means could make him own it,' wrote Morgan; he dressed the ulcer and treated it for a few days. It did not get any better, and the surgeon, 'tould him that I was sure twas veneriall & that he could not be cured without Internalls'. The man consented, and was given a huge dose of purgatives. When he returned, he refused to take the next dose, saying that since the ulcer was half cicatrized already he would not endure such treatment again.[7]

Another venereal patient, a woman, gave Morgan equal pause. She had sores on her arms, had seen many doctors, but to no avail. Morgan dressed her sores, but they did not heal. He wrote, 'after a grate many quivications and Mental resarvations to no purpose I plainly tould her she had or was poxed she semed very angrey at such plain deling in the beginning but at last consented.'[8] She then revealed that she had already been treated two years previously by salivation, but had not mentioned it to Morgan because she had thought herself cured. Venereal disease probably represents the most telling incidence of the negotiations that characterized doctor–patient relationships. It was common, and cures even commoner; either of these two patients could have purchased at least a dozen patent remedies in Bristol itself, or could have sent away for advice or remedies by post. One Bristol surgeon went so far as to have a special side door into an alley for patients with the pox who did not wish to be seen consulting him.[9] But the style of these two interactions was typical of Morgan's practice, even for more obscure or mundane ailments, and highlights the role of the client in shaping medical encounters. As a Bristol medical student in London was advised, 'give early Relief to your Patient and it will be a means of gaining his confidence and esteem, then attack the Disease more radically'.[10]

Thus far, I have relied upon Alexander Morgan, treating his text as a palimpsest, claiming that patients' voices can be discerned through it. Patients' voices can be heard more directly in a variety of sources; some of the best are autobiographies. For the Bristol area, artisans' autobiographies are few in number and varied in purpose. Some authors wrote for religious reasons and published their work, while others wrote in old age for their grandchildren. But in almost all cases, the way in which a person recounts an incident of illness to his reader and to a doctor are the same. In other words, these are not just narratives about illness. They are how illness itself was constituted, for both patient and practitioner.

These tales of illness are striking to the modern reader because they emphasize both the ultimate and the precipitant causes of illness; almost all discussions consider events over a considerable period of time. For the patient, this deeply historical perception of disease had several functions. First, recounting how they fell ill enabled patients to understand their bouts of sickness, to make sense of the seemingly random incidence of disease. For example, this is what Samuel Sholl, a poor silkweaver, recounted in his autobiography:

> my bedfellow scratched my right leg with his toenail; being young and unacquainted with anything of this kind, I did not attend to it; it festered and became so bad that I was obliged to apply to different surgeons, but all in vain, indeed, I was apprehensive it must be cut off; however, as I knew something of medicine, I set about trying some means myself, and I have every reason to be thankful that it answered the end. I cured it, to my unspeakable joy, in about four months, after its being bad between eight and nine years.[11]

For Sholl, this was a tale of resourcefulness. He wanted to emphasize that he was young and knew nothing or the initial scratch would have been better seen to. But with more advanced years and wisdom, Sholl was able to understand his illness, and even to cure himself, when his surgeons had more drastic remedies in mind. Sholl reiterated this theme of youthful ignorance in a visit to a surgeon for painful mouth ulcers. He started his narrative with a snowball fight that had happened when he was a boy, sixteen years earlier. Having been hit in the face with a snowball, he reasoned, was the underlying or initiating cause of his ulcers.[12] This tale of unintended consequences and youthful innocence can be read on many levels. For Sholl, brought up in a prayerful and devout household, the motifs of innocence, fall, and redemption, error and salvation, provided a familiar narrative structure with which to understand what had befallen him.

There were many ways to interpret illness in early modern England, but one of the most common was to put it into this paradigm of careless action. Again and again, patients tell how they unwittingly violated one of the canons of popular medicine by subjecting their bodies to unexpected changes in temperature. For instance, James Lackington, a bookseller (whose autobiography was, in part, a thinly disguised diatribe against Methodism), got very ill taking a coach to Bristol. 'I was so very cold, that when I came to the inn where the passengers dined, I went directly to the fire, which struck the cold inward, so that I had but a very narrow escape from death.'[13] Similarly, John Bennett, a Bristol house-carpenter, recounted how, 'being at a house at work in Clifton, it was very hot, and I drank some cold water, then I was laid up for a week with a bad Stummick'.[14] Finally, a Bristol printer's apprentice, Charles Manby Smith, described the illness of his fellow worker:

> he had caught a chill through incautiously bathing while hot and the doctor had warned him that the consequences might be serious, if not fatal, unless he used great caution. As he used none, the admonition became a veracious prophecy; the cold settled upon his lungs, and he soon fell into a rapid decline.[15]

Despite the varied backgrounds and educational experience of these men, all three (and the printer's doctor) saw dire consequences arising from sudden changes in temperature. Doctors, of course, could easily place their patients' anxieties about hot and cold, wet and dry, within a framework of humoural medicine. Although fashions in medical theory came and went, the basic structure of the four humours, with their associated qualities of hot and cold, wet and dry, was retained well into the nineteenth century.

Testimonials, an extremely popular advertising strategy in the eighteenth century, provide another source of patients' narratives. The veracity of some of these puffs is open to question; but whether 'genuine' lived experience or not, these tales followed similar narrative conventions about illness. For instance, Charity Bull, from Chewton Mendip in Somerset, went to the Glastonbury spa during its extremely brief vogue in the early 1750s. (This spa seems to have been the poor man's Bath; it was repeatedly characterized as the resort of poor and middling sorts.) She had had smallpox when a young woman, and, disliking the redness it left in her face, she dipped her head in cold water a few times every day for a whole summer. 'The consequence was, that she got a severe pain in her Head and Jaws, lost most of her Teeth, became short-breathed, and grew Deaf of her Right Ear.' That was fifteen years prior to her spa cure.[16] Again, whether or not Charity Bull was a purely fictitious character, the author of this testimonial adhered to the convention of seeking illness' cause, however remote, in an event widely recognized as dangerous to the health.

When a physician in Bath noted how people had come to be paralysed, the same sorts of explanation were popular. Hot/cold variations accounted for seven cases, accidental poisoning with white lead for three cases, and post-childbirth for two cases.[17] For virtually every case, a distinct causal event was listed.

Hot/cold, wet/dry interpretations of illness have been noted by Andrew Wear in seventeenth-century Puritan letters and diaries, by Cecil Helman in a twentieth-century British practice, as well as in a wide range of anthropologists' accounts of indigenous medical theories.[18] In early modern England, first, such concepts or explanatory strategies were common to patient and doctor alike, albeit with varying theoretical justification. They provided a common ground, a familiar set of concepts within which the meaning and treatment of illness could be discussed. Second, such hot/cold explanations provided a certain measure of control, or at least the illusion of control against the random incidence of illness. Illness had meaning, and it was related to specific historical events in a person's past that could be elucidated, rather than being random misfortune or divine displeasure. Given the widespread belief in hot/cold causation of illness, it was even possible to avoid illness by being careful about temperature changes. In other words, if you were careful and avoided excesses of hot and cold, you might preserve your health in a world beset by frequent sickness and accident.

It might be expected that overtly religious interpretations of illness would have been a useful, and common, explanatory resource. After all, as David Vincent has suggested, artisan autobiographies (the sources for many of these narratives of illness) were modelled upon the earlier genre of spiritual autobiography.[19] Yet most of these narratives rely upon naturalistic, humouralist explanations, coloured by superstition, the residuum of magic belief still strong in popular culture, rather than explicitly theological ones (although, as in the case of Samuel Sholl, religious narratives could provide structural models).

There are two exceptions to this secular style: Quakers and Methodists (both well-represented in Bristol). These writers of spiritual autobiography interpreted illness in ways quite removed from those of their less godly brethren. Quaker narratives of illness of the late seventeenth century and their Methodist counterparts a century later resemble each other strongly. In both cases, the meaning of illness was not invested in its first causes but in its opportunity for the sufferer to exhibit grace.

For instance, a poor housekeeper, Mrs Oddie, was the subject of a biography in the *Arminian Magazine*, edited by John Wesley and an important link among early Methodists. It claimed that, 'she managed a weak and delicate body with admirable prudence; and bore its pain and weakness with steady patience and the resignation to the will of God', without any reference to how she had come to be in such a state.[20] Episodes of illness could be quite unforeseen occasions of grace. For Sampson Staniforth, his wife's asthma turned out to be such an occasion, for he started preaching in their home when she could not go out.[21] Illness, no matter how severe or painful, was God's work, and in some way beneficial to the sufferer.

For these early Methodists, God intervened swiftly and directly in their lives; hence there was little point in puzzling out the reasons for falling ill. Rather, attention was focused in the opposite direction – towards one's eventual meeting with God.

A hallmark of the truly blessed was their early recognition of their final, fatal illness. In a particularly choice phrase, Mrs Oddie was described as 'visibly ripening for glory' a full three months before she died.[22] Indeed, Methodists were supposed to welcome death if it were God's will. Benjamin Wood, for instance, prayed for his family in his class meeting, 'If my death will contribute any thing to their salvation, thy will be done!' Although in perfect health at the time, he was 'attacked in his head, back, bowels and stomach' and was dead in a few days' time.[23] Submission to the Lord's will implied that the causes of his sudden illness were not discussed; nor was the impact of the family's loss of its chief wage earner.

However, these 'enthusiastic' interpretations of illness were exceptional; they provide a counterpoint to far more widely held beliefs, among doctors and patients, about the importance of the causes of illness. Again, the emphasis upon long-term causation was the central interpretative structure in early modern medical thought, popular and professional. It invested illness with meaning for its sufferers, while simultaneously reflecting and shaping the social realities of doctor–patient interactions.

Early in the century, the patient's and the doctor's words are one. It is easy to hear the patient's voice in the doctor's case report, and, in his autobiography, Sholl recounts his tales to us as he reported them to his surgeon. But over the course of the century, this symmetry fades. Doctors begin to sound like doctors, and patients' voices disappear. Listen, for instance, to this narrative, of a farm labourer, as recounted by a mid-century surgeon. Fifteen years prior to the consultation, 'he got a surfeit (so the country people call any sudden alteration of the blood and juices, by drinking cold liquors when they are very hot . . .).'[24] Already the doctor has distanced himself and his concepts of illness from 'the country people'. Or hear this doctor discussing a young man who experienced, 'as he expressed it, a fluttering in the precordial region on the least motion'.[25] Farm labourers did not refer to their chests as 'precordial regions'. The doctor has taken over, commandeered the patient's own words, almost unconsciously interpreting them and replacing them with his own medical equivalents.

By the 1780s, the patient's narrative was no longer the focus of inquiry in the infirmary. Indeed, the patient himself was reduced to 'a dull contented country lad' with a bladder stone, or 'Mary Townsend, aged thirty years, of a dark complexion, disagreeable Mulatto features and emaciated form' who had supposedly 'led a very dissipated life'.[26] Neither person described thus would have been granted interpretative authority over their illness equal to that of the doctor. Their poverty and dependency was read from their physical features (notice how Mary Townsend's 'disagreeable' features served to support the contention of dissipation) and made them unreliable witnesses.

The transition from the patient's narrative to his or her symptoms and signs was not immediate, but consider this description of a boy in hospital:

> His appearance was florid, his complexion clear. He complained of a slight headach and a sore throat. His pulse was full and rather frequent, the tongue white, the tonsils slightly inflamed, the parotid glands were very much enlarged, the bowels were confined, and there was a little oppression about the chest.[27]

By this time (1816) even the sole mention of the patient's perception, 'he complained of a slight headach', was formulaic. Every other descriptive phrase came from the physical examination of the patient. From such details, doctors adduced the patient's diagnosis.

The patient's narrative was replaced by physical diagnosis and post-mortem dissection. The body, the disease, became the focus of the medical gaze, not the patient's version of illness.[28] In Bristol, James Bedingfield, the infirmary apothecary who later became a surgeon, published a book of cases from the hospital in 1816. Of the thirty-four cases who died, all but two were anatomized. Of course, such dissection represents the ultimate denial of the patient's narrative. Living patients were evaluated by respiratory sounds, temperature, pulse, and condition of the oft-drawn blood.

For patients with any sort of respiratory ailments, the sounds of their breathing were noted carefully. Primitive percussion was used: 'on striking the diseased side with the hand, it sounded heavily and obscurely'.[29] A patient with hydrothorax was diagnosed by 'the symptoms of the disease, together with an attentive examination of the chest in the manner directed by Corvisart'.[30]

Temperatures were used as another indicator of the patient's condition. The evidence is poor, and it does not seem that temperatures were taken regularly; rather, they were used occasionally. For instance, Richard Smith, an infirmary surgeon, noted a rise in temperature in a post-surgical case, and, in another surgical case, the patient's temperature was followed from a high of 102° down to 99½° several days later.[31] The pulse was far more important, since it was the primary indicator for bloodletting, the most common therapeutic intervention. It was taken regularly, and both quantity and quality were noted.

Older styles of explanation did not immediately retreat in response to physical diagnosis. A cooper reported to Bedingfield that 'he was first seized with a cold chill since which time he had been labouring under more or less difficulty of breathing'.[32] Another man owed his illness to 'exposure to great heat in a sugarhouse, to which he was not accustomed, and afterwards going into the open air'.[33] In both instances, the juxtaposition of hot and cold lay at the heart of illness, seemingly for doctor and patient alike.

However, what Bedingfield and colleagues wanted was to reduce their patients to logical physical causes and effects. Thus, when a woman's puzzling pattern of respiration was made explicable in post-mortem dissection, Bedingfield could say, 'the appearances which the parts exhibited upon dissection, afforded a satisfactory elucidation of the symptoms which existed during the life of the patient'.[34] In another case, in which he had recounted the patient's own story, Bedingfield also described the sounds made when the chest was percussed, making an analogy with a half-empty cask with thick oleaginous material inside.[35] He counterbalanced the patient's own words with the objective witness of a physical analogy, in which the patient was reduced to a barrel.

Usually the apothecary was careful to distinguish himself as narrator from the patient, using phrases like 'according to her own account' to demarcate the two points of view.[36] In only two cases did the apothecary give his readers extended versions of patients' narratives; both were puzzling and frustrating cases. As Bedingfield put it, 'I have found considerable difficulty in compressing this case; and even in its present abridged state, it will perhaps appear tedious.'[37] Bedingfield, in his attempts to 'compress this case', in his efforts to present himself as an objective narrator, acknowledged some of the tensions inherent in the meeting between working-class patient and middle-class doctor. Within the hospital, patient and doctor did not meet as equals; indeed, the patron–client relationship had become reversed. Patients were dependent upon doctors to admit them and to allow them to remain in hospital. However, they did not passively become the objects of medical inquiry. Thus, Bedingfield's language mirrors both his attempts to attain interpretative authority over the patient's illness and a very real authority over the patient's body.

Indeed, throughout his text, we see Bedingfield wrestling with problems of authority. For instance, one of his patients, a man with some kind of heart disease, left the hospital because he feared that if he died, his body would be dissected.[38] Bristol hospital patients were forbidden by the rules to swear, or gamble on the wards, as in most infirmaries. But doctors were not given absolute sway over patients, who could (and did) appeal to the hospital's Court of Governors. Bedingfield, as the hospital apothecary (he and the matron were the only full-time hospital employees), was a central figure in the discipline and management of patients.

But textual authority threatened to evade Bedingfield's grasp as well. As discussed, the apothecary used rhetorical devices to reduce the impact of the patient's narrative, and to emphasize his own physical findings. However, Bedingfield was not necessarily having difficulty in conveying the sensory impressions of a physical examination in words. Rather, he borrowed the metaphor of the human chest as a barrel from J. N. Corvisart, the Parisian doctor who specialized in diseases of the heart.[39]

The first English translation of Corvisart's major work had been published in 1813, three years prior to Bedingfield's work, and it is probable that Bedingfield attained his knowledge of Parisian diagnostic technique, at least in part, from this work. Corvisart dealt with the diagnosis and treatment of heart problems, emphasizing careful examination and detailed postmortem analysis. Although Paris hospitals were much older and larger than the Bristol Infirmary, Corvisart too occasionally alluded to problems of authority. For example, in the introduction to his book, he emphasized the need for a doctor to understand moral man, lest he be misled by his patient. 'It is thus, that too often placed between truth and falsehood, the credulous, inexperienced, and over confident Physician, has repeatedly found himself the plaything and laughing stock of perfidious men.'[40] On another occasion, Corvisart, like Bedingfield, disparaged a patient's account of illness, saying, 'if we may believe the patient'.[41] Thus, Bedingfield, in using Corvisart's metaphor of the chest as a barrel (which actually originated with Leopold Auenbrugger, the inventor of percussion), was not only clothing himself in the mantle of Parisian medical sophistication, but was also acknowledging the common attempts of hospital doctors to achieve textual and institutional authority.

The language of diagnosis itself served to separate patients and doctors. Within the infirmary, physicians and surgeons increasingly turned to Latinate diagnoses. 'Cough' became '*Tussis*'; 'wound' became '*Vulnus*'; 'leg ulcers' became '*Ulcus cruris*'. Such diagnoses probably reflect surgeons' aping of physicians in attempts to improve their status, but also indicate the hospital's increasing reliance on William Cullen's nosology. By the 1780s and 1790s, many diagnoses in the infirmary records can be fitted into the Edinburgh professor's scheme of disease classification. Ailments like 'cynanche', or 'peripneumonia', virtually pathognomonic of Cullen's theories, appear in the infirmary register. The shift from English to Latin diagnosis happened quickly.[42] In the late 1770s, 70 per cent of all diagnoses were in English, and 19 per cent in Latin (the remainder were diagnoses in one language that lacked any clear equivalent in the other). By the turn of the century, 79 per cent of all diagnoses were in Latin; only 1 per cent were still in English.

Put in local context, this change is all the more alienating. Somerset dialect was rich in words for illness and disability. For instance, it made distinctions among slow continuous pain ('drimmeling'), continuous aching pain ('nagging'), and the restlessness due to illness ('tavering'). Parts of the body had non-standard names, such as 'pook' for stomach. Common small skin ailments such as whitlows or pimples had a couple of dialect names each.[43] Thus, even standard English was a step away from ordinary discussions of illness; the use of Latin underscored the social distance between doctor and patient, emphasizing the doctor's powerful role within the infirmary.

Therapeutics provided the second flank of the attack on the patient's experience. Bristol hospital medicine had long been characterized by bleeding, bleeding, and more bleeding. Joseph Metford, an infirmary surgeon of the 1770s, recounted that Dr John Paul would ask every patient who entered the hospital if he were a Bristol man. If the answer was yes, Paul ordered twenty ounces of blood let. When Metford asked about this unfailing practice, he replied,

> If he is a Bristol man, I know he sits of an evening smoking tobacco and drinking your abominable fat ale; the first thing to be done is to let some of that run out, and then we shall see what else is the matter.[44]

This story may well be apocryphal but its theme is reiterated in numbers of hospital accounts.

Heroic therapy extended to bleeding patients with haemoptysis, the spitting up of blood from the lungs. Bedingfield justified this practice:

> we are often reduced to the alternative of taking blood from the arm or of allowing it to rush from the lungs. Which mode I would enquire is attended with the greater hazard and inconvenience to the patient?[45]

– inconvenience to the staff as well; this therapeutic style was a system of management. It enabled a handful of part-time doctors to administer care in a hospital with 180 beds, sometimes occupied by two patients each.

Neither of the two mainstays of hospital therapy, bleeding and diet, was performed directly by physicians or surgeons. Bloodletting was done by the surgeons' pupils and apprentices. Two pupils from the early nineteenth century wrote brief descriptions of their student days in the infirmary; bloodletting is prominent in each. Henry Alford, a pupil in the early 1820s, described how patients were bled, not just from the arm, but by cupping, and from the temporal artery and jugular vein. He said, 'all these minor operations were performed by the pupils'.[46] He often bled twenty or more patients per day, and reported that the pupils often complained of the expense of having their lancets re-ground: 'I have seen one or two of them strop their lancets on the soles of their boots.'[47]

At the turn of the century, this sanguinary tendency had hardened into therapeutic regime. Quite simply, most patients were put on an anti-phlogistic regimen that featured bleeding, purging, blisters, and a bland diet. Patients' ailments were quickly categorized as resulting from either inflammatory or diminishing processes. Most patients were evidently suffering from inflammatory diatheses; in Bedingfield's collection of cases, anti-phlogistic outweighed phlogistic therapies five to one.

Such either/or therapeutics simplified hospital practice. The 'House Powder' for example, was a standard cathartic powder mixed up in 1:3 proportions of calomel to jalap. The administration of such a purge, in association with bleeding, constituted a ritual of hospital admission. This style of therapy obliterated the patient's account of him- or herself because it relied upon the body's own response. The body served as its own monitor of therapeutic efficacy. For example, in a case of phrenitis, at least 20 oz of blood were taken from the jugular two or three times a day for four to five days. Bedingfield explained that, 'No regard was paid to the quantity taken; an abatement in the violence of the phrenetic symptoms formed the criterion by which the flow of sanguineous fluid was regulated.'[48] To put it another way, the patient's words were not relevant; his or her body spoke instead.

The body manifested its need for bloodletting in the pulse and in the blood itself. The pulse functioned as an indicator of the patient's over- or under-stimulated state. In apoplexy, for example, if it was full and slow, and the patient's head was red, the jugular arteries full, then bleeding was called for. If, on the other hand, the pulse was 'languid' and the body surface cold, it was contraindicated.[49] As for the blood itself, its condition was noted while it was drawn; did it trickle out, or flow? Then it was allowed to sit for a while and examined once it had separated into its constituent parts. If it had a buffy coat, the patient was suffering from an inflammatory process. If not, in Bristol it might still be considered inflammatory.

In other words, therapeutics and diagnosis both emphasized the aspects of illness most removed from the patient's own understanding. Bristol was no centre of medical innovation or learning. Yet in its infirmary, it developed and made use of medical knowledge appropriate to its changing context. Surgeons diminished the importance of the patient's narrative of illness and emphasized physical diagnosis, which served to privilege surgical technique within the hospital and to discipline its patients. This chapter, in essence, has provided a reading of two texts – Alexander Morgan's apprentice notebook and James Bedingfield's compendium of infirmary cases, along with some ancillary illustrations. Both represent moments in the evolution of certain genre. Patients' narrative drew upon a wide range of models and sources, represented a variety of ways of understanding illness, and appeared in several different forms, such as autobiography, case report, and testimonial. In contrast, Bedingfield's genre was written by and for doctors, and drew largely upon the patient's signs and symptoms.

The shift from narrative to history, in which Bedingfield and Morgan each represent rather different moments, was not unique to Bristol medicine. Rather, it reflects the larger transition from a medicine dominated by private practice, in which a range and number of practitioners competed for patients, to a hospital-based medicine more familiar to modern eyes. Apprentice-trained Alexander Morgan never became associated with the infirmary in any capacity, and enjoyed a substantial surgical practice, in time taking on his own apprentices. But his was the last generation that could completely ignore hospital medicine. By Bedingfield's day, almost all surgeons in Bristol were trained in the hospital, and there learned a different style of practice from Morgan's house-to-house travels.

However, just as medical texts evolved, authors adopting different genres and patterns of language, so too did ordinary people's narratives of illness. Such popular texts should not be understood as unwavering tradition, a backdrop against which medical dramas were played out. In other words, although I have dealt here with changes in medical culture, patients' perspectives were changing too. In conclusion, when Thomas Beddoes wrote in 1804 that the poor preferred to consult their neighbours, rather than doctors, 'because they speak to the sick in their own language', he was describing a rather recent historical reality.[50]

Acknowledgements

I am very grateful to David Cantor, Michael Dennis, Malcolm Nicolson, and Charles Rosenberg for their comments on an earlier version of this paper.

Notes

I regret the lack of discussion of several works which came to my attention since the completion of this paper in 1987: Barbara Duden,

Geschichte unter der Haut: Ein Einsacher Artz und seine Patientinnen um 1730, (Stuttgart, 1987); Harold Brody, *Stories of Sickness*, (New Haven, 1987); Thomas Laqueur, 'Bodies, Details, and the Humanitarian Narrative', in Lynn Hunt, ed., *The New Cultural History*, (Berkeley, 1989), 176–204; Gareth Williams, 'The genesis of chronic illness: narrative re-construction', *Sociology of Health and Illness 6* (1984), 175–200; C. Herzlich and J. Pierret, *Illness and Self in Society*, trans. E. Forster, (Baltimor, 1987); Dorothy Porter and Roy Porter, *Patient's Progress: The Dialects of Doctoring in Eighteenth-Century England*, (Cambridge, 1989); A. Kleinman, *Illness Narratives: Suffering, Healing, and the Human Condition*, (New York, 1988); Charles E. Rosenberg, 'Disease in History: Frames and Farmers', *Milbank Quarterly*, *67*, Supp. 1 (1989), 1–15.

1. Wellcome Institute for the History of Medicine, London, Alexander Morgan's casebook (hereafter referred to as Morgan's casebook) ms. 3631, p. ii.
2. Nicholas Jewson, 'Medical knowledge and the patronage system in eighteenth-century England', *Sociology*, 8 (1974), 369–85; 'The disappearance of the sick-man from medical cosmology, 1770–1870', *Sociology*, 10 (1976), 225–44. See also Malcolm Nicolson, 'The metastatic theory of pathogenesis and the professional interests of the eighteenth century physician', *Medical History*, *32* (1988), 277–300.
3. Cecil Helman, '"Feed a cold, starve a fever" – folk models of infection in an English suburban community, and their relation to medical treatments, *Culture, Medicine and Psychiatry*, 2 (1978), 107–37.
4. John Woodward, *To Do the Sick No Harm* (London, 1974). Guenter B. Risse, *Hospital Life in Enlightenment Scotland, Care and Teaching at the Royal Infirmary of Edinburgh* (Cambridge, 1986); Roy Porter 'The gift relation: philanthropy and provincial hospitals in eighteenth-century England', in Lindsay Granshaw and Roy Porter (eds,) *The Hospital in History* (London, 1989).
5. This discussion is drawn from my dissertation, 'The physic of charity: health and welfare in the West Country, 1690–1834', PhD thesis, University of Pennsylvania, 1988.
6. Morgan's casebook, p. 1; see also pp. 17, 61, 95, for further examples.
7. Morgan's casebook, p. 16. On the healers of venereal ailments, see W.F. Bynum, 'Treating the wages of sin: venereal disease and specialism in Eighteenth-century Britain', in W.F. Bynum and Roy Porter (eds.), *Medical Fringe and Medical Orthodoxy* 1750–1850 (London, 1987).
8. Morgan's casebook, p. 18.
9. W. H. Harsant, 'Medical Bristol in the eighteenth century', *Bristol Medico-Chirurgical Journal* (December 1899), 7.
10. University of Bristol Medical School, Broughton lecture notes, UA DM 1H p. 117. See also Adrian Wilson's comments on William Hunter's professional persona in his paper, 'William Hunter and the varieties of man-midwifery', in Roy Porter and William F. Bynum, (eds), *William Hunter and the Eighteenth Century Medical World* (Cambridge, 1985).

11. Samuel Sholl, *A Short Historical Account of the Silk Manufacture in England* (London, 1811), p. 43.
12. Ibid., p. 47.
13. James Lackington, *Memoirs* (London, 1792). p. 130.
14. Bristol Record Office, Bennett ms. autobiography, p. 8.
15. Charles Manby Smith, *The Workingman's Way in the World* . . . (London, n.d.), p. 11.
16. Anon., *'Wilt Thou be Made Whole'* . . . (London, 1751), pp. 21–2.
17. Anon., *Narrative of the Efficacy of Bath Waters* (Bath, 1787).
18. Cecil Helman, '"Feed a cold, starve a fever"'; Andrew Wear, 'Puritan perceptions of illness in seventeenth-century England' in Roy Porter (ed.), *Patients and Practitioners; Lay Perceptions of Medicine in Pre-industrial Society* (Cambridge, 1985). For just one example of this concept in other cultures, see Katherine Gould-Martin, 'Hot cold clean poison and dirt: Chinese folk medical categories', *Social Science and Medicine* 12 (1978), 39–46. See also Charles E. Rosenberg, 'The therapeutic revolution', in the book of the same name, Charles E. Rosenberg and Morris Vogel (eds) (Philadelphia, 1979), for the persistence of such categories in nineteenth-century America.
19. David Vincent, *Bread, Knowledge and Freedom* (London, 1981), pp. 14–19.
20. *Arminian Magazine* (1783), p. 356.
21. *Arminian Magazine* (1783), p. 350.
22. *Arminian Magazine* (1783), p. 357.
23. *Arminian Magazine* (1783), pp. 414–15.
24. Rice Charlton, *Cases of Persons* . . ., (Bath, 1774), p. 6.
25. Marmaduke Berdoe, *An Enquiry into the Influence of the Electrical Fluid in the Structure and Formation of Animated Beings* (Bath, 1771), p. 149.
26. Thomas Beddoes, *On Fever* (Clifton, n.d.), case #21; James Bedingfield, *A Compendium of Cases from the Bristol Infirmary* (London, 1816), p. 155.
27. James Bedingfield, *A Compendium of Medical Practice* (London, 1816), p. 6.
28. Obviously, I draw upon Michel Foucault, *The Birth of the Clinic*, trans. A. Sheridan (New York, 1973), in focusing upon doctors' new ways of perceiving the body. But Foucault's epistemic shift was not sudden; rather it derived from the changing social realities within hospitals, be they French or English.
29. Bedingfield, *A Compendium of Cases*, p. 116.
30. Ibid., p. 125.
31. Beddoes, *On Fever*.
32. Bedingfield, *A Compendium of Cases*, p. 146.
33. Ibid., p. 94.
34. Ibid., p. 83.
35. Ibid., p. 115.
36. Ibid., p. 89, for this example.
37. Ibid., pp. 114–16.
38. Ibid., pp. 147–8.

39. Corvisart actually disparaged the analogy of the chest as a barrel, but it is difficult to know where else Bedingfield (who cites Corvisart) might have found this figure of speech. Leopold Auenbrugger, the inventor of percussion, used this metaphor, but his work had not yet been translated into English, and about the only English review of his work (which Bedingfield was unlikely to have seen) compared the chest to a drum, rather than a barrel (see Saul Jarcho, 'A review of Auenbrugger's Inventum Novum', *Bulletin of the History of Medicine*, 33 (1959), 470–4).

40. J. N. Corvisart, *A Treatise on the Diseases of the Heart and Great Vessels*, trans. C. H. Hebb (London, 1813), p. xi.

41. Ibid., pp. 286–7.

42. This analysis is based upon a sample of 1024 infirmary patients, 1770–1805, from the registers of in- and out-patients at the Bristol Infirmary, Bristol Record Office, 35893 19, 20.

43. W. P. Williams, and W. A. Jones, 'A list of Somerset dialect', *Somerset Archaeological and Natural History Society Proceedings* 18 (1871).

44. Bristol Record Office, Biographical Memoirs, vol. 2, p. 1012.

45. Bedingfield, *A Compendium of Cases*, p. 39.

46. Henry Alford, 'The Bristol Infirmary in my student days 1822–28', *Bristol Medico-Chirurgical Journal* (September 1890), 189.

47. Ibid., p. 190.

48. Bedingfield, *A Compendium of Cases*, p. 37.

49. Ibid., p. 29.

50. Thomas Beddoes, *Rules of the Preventive Medical Institution*, (Bristol, 1804), p. 94. I am very grateful to Mrs Dorothy Stansfield, Beddoes's most recent biographer, for calling this quotation to my attention.

5

Robert Carswell and William Thomson at the Hôtel-Dieu of Lyons: Scottish views of French medicine

Stephen Jacyna

Introduction

In the decades after 1815 France was the unquestioned world centre for western medicine. Students flocked there not only from other European nations but also from North America to learn the latest doctrines and, to be trained in the most modern techniques. This phenomenon has attracted much attention from historians concerned with such issues as national styles in medicine and in the transfer of knowledge and technologies. In particular, Russell Maulitz has analysed the attraction of French medicine for British students, while John Harley Warner has examined the way in which the French experience was represented by American students upon their return to their native land.[1]

These studies have both tended towards a similar conclusion: that the relations between French medicine and those of other nations cannot be conceived as a process of simple osmosis whereby the knowledge offered by the host nation was passively assimilated by these visitors and later deployed in their home context. On the contrary, the transfer of knowledge was throughout characterized by the selection, interpretation, and adaptation by these foreign students of what they found in France. This modification of the foreign import was determined by domestic considerations; to understand fully the role of France in early nineteenth-century medicine it is therefore necessary to adopt a dual perspective. It is not sufficient to ask only what the donor nation had to *offer*: the historian must also consider what the recipient *required*.

The present chapter is intended to contribute to an understanding of this interplay between supply and demand in early nineteenth-century medicine. It adopts a somewhat different viewpoint from earlier studies. Whereas these have taken a 'macro' approach to the question – making whole populations of students the object of enquiry – I propose to select a much higher power of magnification and focus on two individuals. Something is clearly lost by adopting this micro perspective. In particular, all efforts to generalize from it are fraught with difficulty. Something new and valuable is, however, gained: first, a much more immediate notion of what it was *like* to be a foreign medical student in France; and, second, an account of the experience that has not been edited for publication or modified to suit a particular audience or polemical purpose. Given such materials it is possible to derive additional insights into the issues of why such students flocked to France, how they viewed the practices of their hosts, and what they derived from these medical pilgrimages.

The actors: Robert Carswell and William Thomson

A study of this kind is dependent upon the survival of sources of a particular character. Fortunately, a group of some of the most prominent channel-crossers have left large caches of documents relating to their time in France. These were the individuals who went to France at the instigation of John Thomson (1765–1846); they included his two sons, William and Allen Thomson (1802–52; 1809–84), and Robert Carswell (1793–1857), a close associate of the Thomson family. All three were eventually to hold chairs in British universities.

John Thomson (1765–1846) is best known as the biographer of Cullen and as the first holder of the Chair of Pathology in Edinburgh. He was a key figure in the development of pathological and surgical teaching in Edinburgh in the first three decades of the nineteenth century; in particular, he introduced many of the newest Continental ideas to his medical brethren.

Maulitz has also remarked upon Thomson's pivotal role in encouraging Edinburgh students to pursue further studies in France.[2] William Thomson and Carswell were, however, distinguished from these others by the particular purpose attached to their Continental journeys: the collection of pathological data – and, above all, pathological *illustrations* – to be used in John Thomson's teaching in Edinburgh.

The most tangible residue of this grand design are collections of documents in Edinburgh, Glasgow, and London recording the efforts of the Thomsons and their helpers to achieve these goals.[3] In particular, Edinburgh University Library possesses a collection of manuscripts which, although attributed solely to Carswell, in fact contains contributions from all the major and some minor participants in this endeavour.[4]

A large part of this collection is derived from Carswell and William Thomson's French expeditions. They spent most of their time at the major Parisian hospitals, but also visited a number of provincial centres. In particular, they spent several months in late 1823 and early 1824 at the Hôtel-Dieu of Lyons. It is this aspect of their French experience that provides the focus of this chapter. There are two principal reasons for this selection. In the first place, it is salutary to be reminded that, despite the predominance of Paris, there were other centres of attraction in France for foreign students. Second, in terms both of its style and its content, the Lyons record stands apart from the notes that they made while in Paris. The numerous hospitals in which Thomson and Carswell worked tend in the Parisian portion of their notes to appear merely as names under which sets of autopsy and clinical observations are collected. The institutions themselves and the individuals who worked within them are scarcely characterized. In contrast, the Lyons record provides a vivid and unified account of Carswell's and Thomson's interaction with and reaction to one French hospital and its medical practitioners.

The setting: L'Hôtel-Dieu de Lyon

Carswell and Thomson came to Lyons little more than two years after a School of Medicine based upon the Hôtel-Dieu and Charité hospitals had been created there by royal decree.[5] Some form of medical instruction had, however, been offered in Lyons for many years prior to the formal inauguration of the school. In particular, *surgery* had been taught at the Hôtel-Dieu continuously since 1792.[6] The prime mover in the establishment of the Lyons school of surgery in the post-revolutionary period was Marc Antoine Petit. He was one of the most distinguished of Desault's students, and sought to establish in Lyons a centre of surgical instruction on the model established by his master at the Hôtel-Dieu of Paris.[7]

This strong surgical bias was especially significant for what William Thomson was to derive from his time in Lyons. The availability of extensive opportunities for surgical instruction there appears to have been the chief attraction of the Hôtel-Dieu for him. Although there had been a Chair of Clinical Surgery in Edinburgh since 1803, the incumbent, James Russell, was not a stimulating teacher. Some clinical teaching had been conducted by the surgeons-in-ordinary at the Royal Infirmary since the eighteenth century; however, this remained a department of medical education in which Edinburgh was deficient.[8] There are, moreover, indications that, even in Paris, the surgical training available to Thomson had severe limitations.[9]

The existence of an academic school of medicine in Lyons seems to have impinged little upon Carswell's and Thomson's activities. Thomson dutifully listed all the courses on offer, but there is nothing to indicate that either he or his companion attended any of them.[10] By the time he came to France, Thomson had received a pretty full academic medical education (see Table 5.1). It is not possible to be as certain of Carswell's prior education: while he appears to have taken only the anatomy course in Edinburgh, he did study medicine for a time in Glasgow. In any case, it was what they could learn on the wards and the dead-room of the Hôtel-Dieu, rather than in its lecture theatres, that appears to have attracted most of the attention of the two visitors.

William Thomson, did, however, show an interest in the institution as a whole, making notes on the architecture, organization, and logistics of the hospital. These were intended to form part of a larger account of the hospitals he visited on the Continent; however, the notebook on 'Foreign Hospitals' to which he on one occasion refers does not appear to have survived.[11]

Thomson's description of the Hôtel Dieu provides a valuable snapshot of a French provincial hospital in 1823–4. Its true interest lies, however, in the fact that it illuminates which aspects of this setting attracted Thomson's attention and, in

Table 5.1 William Thomson's medical education prior to 1822 (Reconstructed from Edinburgh University Matriculation Rolls)*

1818–19: Anatomy, mathematics II.
1819–20: *Possibly* chemistry *or* logic.
A William Thomson of Edinburgh also took John Thomson's course in military surgery in this year.
1820–21: Practice of medicine. *Possibly* materia medica and clinical medicine.

*The interpretation of the Matriculation Rolls is complicated by the fact that more than one William Thomson is listed in each of the relevant years. In some cases the student's place of origin is given: 'William Thomson of Edinburgh' can usually be assumed to be the Thomson in question. In 1820–1 there are, however, *two* William Thomsons of Edinburgh; in consequence, it is unclear how many courses the Thomson in question took.

some instances, reveals his reactions and attitudes to what he saw. It can thus tell as much about the *observer* as about what he witnessed.

Thomson described the fabric of the wards, how patients were distributed between them, and how they were furnished. No detail seemed too small to warrant mention: he reported that 'The beds are of iron – They are provided with curtains and according to the french custom there are two mattrasses [sic] in each. The beds are not two passages distant from one another and the intermediate passage not more than six feet.'[12]

On occasion, simple description is supplemented by evaluation and, indeed, criticism. Thus Thomson noted that 'The beds seem by no means secured against vermin – In taking down the bandages of a fractured thigh which had remained for a *considerable* time untouched I have seen (25th Sept) the bugs crawl forth in swarms so that the Surgeon could not proceed with his examination – I saw people today engaged in burning wound [sic] round the joints of the beds.'[13] French prodigality, as well as their slovenly hygiene, also attracted disapproval. 'In following the Surgical visit it is impossible not to be struck by the useless waste of linen that takes place. Sponges being in no case used for the dressing of wounds.'[14]

In general, Thomson approached the organization of the Hôtel-Dieu not with mere curiosity, but with clear criteria of how a hospital should be run by which he *judged* what he saw. This attitude is indicative of a self-assurance in the face of French practices that was still more apparent in his and Carswell's reactions to the medical and surgical procedures they witnessed.

This interest in the minutiae of hospital organization is another instance of the way in which domestic concerns were reflected in reporting the foreign experience. Controversy had raged in Edinburgh in 1818 over defects in the management of the Royal Infirmary, and John Thomson had issued two pamphlets condemning the current regime.[15]

The primary focus of attention in Thomson's account of the Hôtel-Dieu was not the details of patient care, but the social organization of the hospital. He recorded the numbers of the nursing staff, distinguishing between the 'soeurs' and 'frères' in the service of the Hôtel-Dieu, and subdivided these to show the numbers of fully ordained and novice members. He had also obtained figures showing the numbers of religious at the hospital in 1812 and noted these to show how the nursing staff had increased. The sisters, Thomson noted, received 30 francs a year and the brothers 40, as well as their food and clothing. The hospital also employed fifteen '*hommes de peine*' – presumably to perform heavy work.[16]

Nursing by members of religious orders might be expected to be something to excite the curiosity of a visitor from a Protestant nation. However, Thomson had already seen much of this in the Parisian hospitals; and, after giving these figures, he shifted his attention to the medical staff.

Thomson detailed the number and mode of appointment of the hospital's physicians; the times at which they made their rounds; and the fact that they were always accompanied by their clerk and two nurses. One of these (as well as the clerk) took down prescriptions, while the other hung up tickets indicating diet, blisters, and other forms of treatment. During their visits, Thomson remarked, the physicians 'are dressed in a large black professor's gown'.[17]

It was, however, the surgical service of the Hôtel-Dieu that received closest scrutiny. Thomson gave a detailed account of the ranks of the surgeons and the conditions under which they held their appointments. The surgical wards were in the charge of a 'Surgeon-Major' and an 'aide-major'. The latter remained in post for six years when he then became Surgeon-Major – which post he could hold for a further six years. Both these surgeons were prohibited from marrying.[18]

It is likely that Thomson was sensitized to such questions of the appointment and conditions of surgical staff by the bitter disputes that had raged in Edinburgh in the early nineteenth century over the organization of the surgical service to the Royal Infirmary.[19] John Thomson had been one of the protagonists in these conflicts, and, even in 1823, the issues raised were far from fully resolved. Given this background, it is easily understood why William Thomson should find how other institutions handled such matters a topic of particular interest.

As well as this retrospective motive, Thomson was probably looking to his own future in scrutinizing the way surgery was organized at the Hôtel-Dieu. A new system of surgical attendance at the Royal Infirmary had been introduced in 1818 by which an assistant-surgeoncy fell vacant every other year.[20] The possibility of obtaining one of these posts when he returned to Edinburgh may have spurred Thomson to learn as much as possible of the practice and organization of surgery in a foreign hospital. In the event, upon his return be became one of the surgeons to the New Town Dispensary.

Thomson also noted the existence of a class of '10 young men styled Chirurgiens Internes' at the Hôtel-Dieu. These corresponded roughly to the six surgical dressers who attended the Royal Infirmary; there appear, however, to have been significant differences in their responsibilities and relations to the senior staff. Thomson was struck by the degree of discretion allowed to the Internes in the choice of applications; indeed, he felt that they were given *too* much freedom in this direction. On the other hand, whereas the dressers at the Royal Infirmary performed many simple operations themselves, in Lyons, 'with the exception of bleeding M. Mortier [the aide-major] seems to perform every surgical operation himself opening even the simplest abscesses with his own hands'.[21]

Not only the distribution of responsibilities but also the social relationship between junior and senior surgeons attracted Thomson's notice. He remarked upon the 'Freedom with which the Internes are chided by their superiors'. One wretched Interne was, on 1 October 1823, addressed by the Surgeon-Major, Louis Janson (1787–1870) in Thomson's hearing as 'Bête que vous êtes'.[22]

These remarks – and Thomson's account of the Hôtel-Dieu in general – need to be seen against the background of the instability and self-criticism prevalent in contemporary Edinburgh medicine.[23] In these debates foreign models served to supply alternatives to the established ways that were now under scrutiny. Thomson's account of the Hôtel-Dieu of Lyons – warts and all – is an interesting contrast to the numerous invocations of French practices that figure in this controversial literature. John Thomson, for example, was especially fond of turning to France for resources to criticize aspects of Edinburgh medicine to which he objected and for models of how medical teaching and practice *should* be organized.

His son's account was, in contrast, written, as far as can be judged, for his own benefit, had he ever published it no doubt the polemical interests that agitated his father would have influenced the representation of his immediate impressions. His extant remarks offer a more authentic picture of how an Edinburgh-trained practitioner viewed the French institutions. Instead of an idealized picture, slanted to support some prior contention, they reveal a dispassionate, evaluative, and often critical attitude to what Thomson encountered. While he was ready to learn from the French, he was by no means in awe of them. Moreover, the same presumptions that informed Thomson's remarks on the organization of the Hôtel-Dieu are also evident in what he and Carswell had to say about its clinical practices.

The most numerous of the hospital's inhabitants – the patients – figure little in the notes. Except on a few occasions neither Carswell nor Thomson bothered to record the names of the individuals whose cases attracted their attention. They generally left a space to enter a note of the person's age; on many occasions, however, this remains blank. If any description is given of the patient's own account of his or her symptoms, it tends to be sketchy: there is no attempt to record a comprehensive case history.

The general impression given by the Lyons manuscript – and this is also typical of their Parisian notes – is that Carswell and Thomson were interested in patients not as individuals but as the loci of disease. Moreover, the patient's words were not even of primary importance in establishing the character of that disease. Physical examination completed by autopsy was, in the majority of cases, adequate.

There are, however, exceptions where some peculiarity of the patient's biography seemed sufficiently interesting to warrant mention. Thus on two occasions it is recorded that the patient had served in the French army during the Napoleonic Wars. In the first of these the significance of this fact is not clear. Thomson merely remarks that on 17 October 1823 he and

Carswell were present at the autopsy of a man who had died from dropsy who 'had served upwards of 30 years in the army and had been with the French army in Egypt'.[24] In the second case there is an explicit connection between the patient's military career and his current complaint. This was a man with an intractable ulcer on the nose; Thomson notes that 'The patient states that he received a small sabre-cut upon the nose at the battle of Austerlitz which never healed up completely'.[25] Thomson's special interest in these cases can, once again, be referred to his background: he was the son of a former Professor of Military Surgery in Edinburgh who had helped tend the wounded after Waterloo.

The relation between a patient's occupation or life-style and the aetiology of his condition earns occasional mention elsewhere in the manuscript. Lyons was one of the earliest centres of industrialization in France, with a large proportion of the population engaged in the manufacture of silk. Only one case is, however, related to these social conditions; this was one 'P. Claude. 11 years of age, weaver of Silk, Lyons. This young boy occupied in a work to which his strength was not adequate, had a rhume violent 6 months ago, to which there continued a cough.'[26]

Another record makes it clear that the Hôtel-Dieu served a rural as well as an urban population. Carswell drew the leg ulcers of a wood-cutter who stated that 'previous to his limb becoming affected he had been in the habit of sleeping in the woods upon straw without further shelter both summer and winter and that during the latter season he frequently found himself covered with a thick layer of Snow'. He had been in the hospital in 1822 and had left cured: 'The ulcers however broke out again whilst he was walking homewards – a distance of 22 leagues.'[27]

What makes the paucity and poverty of the patient records all the more noteworthy is that Thomson and Carswell *did*, very rarely, display extended conceptions of what was relevant and important and show that they possessed protocols for recording this information. They appear, however, to have resorted to this extended form of case history only with patients whose circumstances were peculiar to the point of being bizarre.

The fullest of Carswell's case reports is of 'Francois Carveillier [?] aged 63. Porter, biliosanguinary temperament, of a wise well regulated conduct.' Despite the latter trait, he was

> engaged by one of his friends to dinner and drank more than was his custom, which made him tumble in returning home, in which his face was bruised.
>
> Since that accident he has suffered violent pains of the Head, and experienced a difficulty of expressing himself and lost entirely memory. He performed his customary labour with the greatest difficulty.
>
> His state becoming worse from day to day he determined, two months after the accident, to enter the Hôtel-Dieu de Lyon where he was not received. The persons with whom he lived seeing him really unwell, notwithstanding the refusal of the Surgeon, undertook to produce him a fever which could not be doubted, or to make him eat and drink much which would have the desired effect. He presented himself in a state of stupor accompanied with great fever and was then admitted[.]

There then follows a description of this patient's symptoms on admission, the treatment administered, the changes that occurred in his condition, and finally the results of the autopsy that followed his death.[28] Besides the strange story of his admission, there is nothing to indicate why this case should have warranted such special attention.

On two occasions Carswell and Thomson break into their ritual note-taking to recount extraordinary incidents that had occurred on the wards. Thomson began the record of a man who entered the hospital with gunshot wounds of the legs; after a routine description of his injuries and treatment he tells how on going into the ward

> this morning . . . about 10 O'Clock I found this man in the bath, where two soeurs and two men were holding him. He was moving as if he wished to get out and M. Janson who happened to pass seemed to think he had some apprehension of the water as he desired that a cloth should be thrown before him. His struggles or convulsions still continued however, a spumous foam began to issue from his mouth & as the assistants were attempting to raise him out of the bath, he expired in their arms, in a state Mr Carswell thought of asphyxia.[29]

This record is of interest because it shows that, although they kept separate notes, Thomson and Carswell on occasion toured the hospital jointly.

Carswell himself detailed a case which was remarkable because the patient's behaviour while in the hospital was held to shed light on the origins of the condition that had brought him there. A 22-year-old man was admitted with some ulcers on his penis; his disease was judged to be scrofulous, not venereal. However,

> The Clerc who dressed him, found him frequently, if not always in erection at the time he dressed him and observing occasionally drops of blood on his shirt and on the penis or scrotum – When asked from whence it proceeded, he said leeches had been applied to the lower parts; which was not true. From these circumstances the Clerc suspected that he was in the habit of indulging to an excessive degree a venerial [sic] appetite, which had produced the disease of the Testicles and penis.[30]

Carswell succeeded in discovering anatomical corroboration for what had been suspected from the patient's behaviour. When 'the external form of his Cranium was examined . . . the posterior part of it was found to be remarkably prominent. After death, the Cerebellum was found to be nearly twice its usual size and very firm.'[31] In the craniological system of Gall and Spurzheim, which was hotly contested in Edinburgh,[32] the cerebellum was the organ of amativeness.

On most other occasions when the patient appears as an active agent, rather than as the passive bearer of disease, he is also seen as culpable, if not for his condition, then for the unhappy outcome of his treatment. On no less than five occasions a deterioration in a patient's condition – or even his death – is ascribed to a wilful violation of the diet prescribed by the physician or surgeon. Visiting friends and relatives bearing unauthorized foodstuffs were accessories to these infractions.[33]

On the whole, therefore, Carswell and Thomson presented a 'doctor-centred' rather than a 'patient-centred' view of the Hôtel-Dieu. Patients figure only as the sometimes rebellious seats of the diseases that the medical staff must study and tend. It is these diseases and the modes of treatment adopted by the surgeons and physicians of the hospital that form the core of the manuscript.

Carswell at the Hôtel-Dieu: the primacy of pathology

Carswell and Thomson went to France with a common purpose: the execution of John Thomson's commission to gather pathological data and illustrations. The Carswell papers show that, while in Paris, they pursued this goal with great single-mindedness. The record of their visit to Lyons reveals, however, the beginnings of a divergence of interest.

Carswell remained faithful to the original intention of the mission. He was not oblivious to the details of clinical practice that he necessarily witnessed while present in the wards of the Hôtel-Dieu, nor did he refrain from commenting on them when he saw occasion. These comments show the same self-assurance that Thomson exhibited when discussing French methods. Sometimes Carswell's judgement was positive: he could remark in passing that an operation he attended 'was performed by M. Mortier with great dexterity and accuracy'.[34] It could also be critical, ranging from an implicit rebuke to a withering denunciation. Early on in his time in Lyons Carswell came upon a 'young man about 17 years of age [who] was brought into the hospital from the country from a distance of several leagues' with his foot connected to the leg only by tendon and muscle and in a state of extreme gangrene. In this condition, 'he was allowed to remain without an operation for nearly a week!!! at the expiration of which time the constitutional symptoms had increased considerably'. Carswell concluded that the 'negligence of Mr Janson in this case was evidently criminal'.[35]

Whether his judgement was or was not favourable, the clinical aspect of the case was, however, incidental to Carswell; these details came to his notice while he pursued his true, pathological interests. Despite his obvious outrage at what he saw as patent malpractice in the above case, once the gangrenous leg *was* amputated, Carswell's attention switched away entirely from the patient – whose ultimate fate is not described – to the dismembered limb. He lamented the fact that 'What were [sic] the diseased state of the several parts of the leg etc. I am sorry I have been unable to learn anything, having been confined at the time – and the Leg not having been examined on account of its extremely bad smell!!!' Disapproval at clinical incompetence was replaced by annoyance that an opportunity to study disease had been wasted.

This rapid switch of attention can be seen as an illustration of what Maulitz has called the 'synergy' between clinical medicine and pathology in the early nineteenth century. During this period, he writes, the physicians 'who made their daily rounds and attended patients at the bedside were the same as those who tested the boundaries of knowledge about pathological anatomy. . . . In the medical mind of the 1810s and 1820s, pathology was linked inextricably with a series of central problems of clinical medicine.'[36]

There are plentiful instances of this intimacy between clinical and pathological concerns in Carswell's notes. Thus in the case of the 11-year-old silk-weaver mentioned above Carswell frequently employed the stethoscope in an attempt to diagnose the condition prior to death and then sought to confirm his suppositions at autopsy.[37]

However, the close correlation of clinical and pathological concerns is most strikingly apparent in a case of 'cancer of the eye' which Carswell discusses at length. He examined the patient on admission and made a note of her symptoms – especially the headaches she experienced. He attended the operation for the extirpation of the eye, which was 'performed well and expeditiously'. He then subjected the eye to close examination: this revealed that the 'disease, which while the eye was in situ seemed to have *no defined boundary*, was now seen to *adhere only* to the *cornea* and a *small* part of the *conjunctiva*'. Section showed that the cornea, although attached to the tumour, was of its natural structure, and the other parts of the eye were completely healthy.[38]

Carswell proceeded to draw out the implications of these discoveries for future practice. 'From the state of the eye and its appendages,' he wrote,

> which the Pathological Anatomy of the case has shewn were in a perfectly health condition except the Cornea, it appears almost that a simple and partial operation would have been sufficient for the complete extirpation of this affection. Had I previous to the operation, examined the

> eye with more care, and found that the Disease consisted of a tumour having such a limited attachment to its anterior surface . . . I would have been almost certain that the disease was not [this word is crossed out in the original; from the context, however, it must stand] of a cancerous nature; that it was external to the Eye, and that it was not a case of Fungus Haematodes as I suspected. That it was not the latter disease might have been presumed from the age of the patient and also perhaps from the manner in which it had commenced [following trauma].

The nature of the headaches accompanying benign and malignant tumours of the eye might also, Carswell concluded, be of value in differentiating between the two.[39] There could hardly be clearer evidence of the interchangeability of the roles of pathologist and clinician.

A careful reading of Carswell's autopsy reports reveals, however, other concerns which conform less well to this model. As well as his attention to clinico-pathological correlations, Carswell displayed a marked interest in what might be called 'pure' pathology. In other words, he sought in the bodies he dissected the means to an enhanced understanding of disease.

This interest was sometimes expressed in Carswell's alertness to appearances similar to those he had encountered previously and which might represent a 'typical' form of disease.[40] However, this was not merely a natural-historical curiosity in 'interesting' specimens: from such recurring forms Carswell sought to derive general pathological *principles*. Thus, while describing a hernia, he notes that 'in several cases of this kind which I have seen the peritoneum was always formed into cysts, within which the protruding epiploon was lodged. . . . It is probable that the greater number of epiploic herniae which take place in this situation are encysted.' He went on to consider the likely manner in which these cysts were formed.[41] Other processes which received similar treatment included: the anatomical nidus of tubercular ulcers of the intestine;[42] the ossification of the arterial system in senile gangrene;[43] and the cerebral lesions accompanying delirium and fever.[44]

One topic in particular drew Carswell's attention: the manner in which disease and its products spread from one tissue or organ to another. He gave an extended account of an ulcer on the peritoneum in a case of cancer of the stomach because it supplied 'as fine an example as may be met with, of the propagation of that diseased action which produces the cancerous degeneration of one tissue, to another separately from the primitive seat of disease by parts in all appearances healthy, and their subsequent union after a lapse of time'.[45]

In another instance Carswell noted the presence of a white cerebriform matter in some blood vessels in the neighbourhood of a diseased bladder. This observation led him to ask

> How did [these vessels] become filled with the cerebriform matter which formed the fungus excrescences and into which they penetrated? Did it depend on a vital process or simply on mechanical agency? That is had the arteries absorbed this matter or was it forced into them by pressure produced during the violent contraction of the bladder necessary to overcome the resistance which the enlarged prostate presented to the exit of the urine?[46]

Such speculations illustrate a theoretical vein that runs through Carswell's notes. His interest was not only to make observations bearing directly on clinical issues; he strove to uncover something of the processes at work in the body during disease.

Carswell's Lyons notes provide an insight into the ambivalent status of pathology in the 1820s. It remained institutionally and, to a great degree, cognitively dependent upon clinical medicine. At the same time, however, pathology was beginning to acquire a set of research goals distinct from the concerns of the clinic, but closely related to those of the physiologist. Carswell's autopsy reports reveal both the persistence of the clinician-pathologist and the glimmerings of an autonomous science of pathology.

Thomson at the Hôtel-Dieu: the scientific surgeon

William Thomson also spent time in the dead-house of the Hôtel-Dieu and in the preparation of pathological specimens. Only rarely, however, did he show an interest in pathological phenomena in their own right; usually his attention was firmly fixed upon questions relevant to clinical practice.

Thomson's attention at autopsies was, fixed upon matters

of significance to the practice of surgery. On 19 September 1823 he was present at the dissection of a man who had been operated upon some ten days earlier for calculus of the bladder. At the operation the surgeon Mortier suspected that not all the stones had been removed although he could detect none either with the sound or through the wound. The autopsy served to confirm this suspicion when an additional calculus was discovered high up in the bladder. It also revealed that the prostate was much enlarged – something that Mortier had not suspected prior to the operation.[47]

Some of Thomson's accounts of such autopsies are revealing of the attitudes of the French surgeons to these procedures. On occasion they seem to have served as opportunities for the demonstration of the surgeon's ability to *predict* what would be found upon opening the body on the basis of what had been observed during life. Thus, prior to opening the body of a boy who had died after fracturing his leg, 'M. Mortier expressed his opinion that we should find marks of Gastro-Enterité [sic] the consequence of three different excesses of diet of which he had been guilty and the symptoms of which he conceived had returned after each excess.' In fact, the autopsy provided little evidence to support this conjecture; Mortier was obliged to resort to considerable ingenuity in interpreting what was found in order to save his hypothesis.[48]

There is an element of bravado in such displays of diagnostic acumen. In this instance, a special motive of wishing to place the responsibility for his death upon the patient himself can also be inferred. It is likely, moreover, that this particular prediction had a further significance: according to the system of Broussais, which was then at the height of its popularity, inflammation of the gastro-intestinal tract was the lesion that underlay all febrile disorders. There is a hint elsewhere in the manuscript that Mortier was an adherent of this system.[49] This autopsy appears to have served as an attempt to vindicate a prior theoretical commitment.

Thomson was not content with what he could learn about surgery at the Hôtel-Dieu in the autopsy room. To a far greater extent than Carswell, his notes reveal regular and assiduous attendance upon the surgical wards and at operations; while Carswell's interest in clinical matters was subordinate to his pathological investigations, with Thomson the converse was the case.

He appears to have attached himself to Mortier and followed his surgical service closely. Certain topics Thomson found of special interest. Mortier's methods in the treatment of fractures received particular attention. The practical bent and minute detail of these observations is striking: nothing appeared too trivial to warrant recording. Thomson remarked, for example, that 'The beds at the hotel [sic] Dieu are too soft for cases of fracture so that M. Mortier complained there is a valley at one place and mountains at another.' Thomson concluded that 'The bedsteads ought to be higher so that only one instead of two mattresses should be required to bring the patient to the proper level.'[50]

Mortier's method of dressing various fractures came under close scrutiny. Thomson devoted a great deal of space, for instance, to explaining precisely how Mortier applied a simplified version of Desault's apparatus to a fractured clavicle.[51] Mortier's various dicta and rules of thumb in such matters are also faithfully recorded: when an 80-year-old man with a broken femur entered the hospital the French surgeon 'contented himself with placing the limb in a state of demiflexion by placing cushions below the ham alleging that when splints are applied to persons at this advanced period of life they are very liable to cut their way into the muscles'.[52] From these remarks, emerges an image of surgery as a craft, to be learned by apprenticeship.

Thomson was, however, far from being a mere surgical novice dutifully recording the wisdom of a master. He showed on this, as on other occasions, a confidence in his own judgement and ability to *evaluate* rather than merely describe what he saw. At the conclusion of his report of the treatment of compound fractures at the Hôtel-Dieu he commented:

> It appears to me that M. Mortier meddles too much with the wound for the purpose of pressing out pus and cleaning its surface as he almost constantly occasions more or less haemorrhage. It appears to me too that in the present irritable state of the wound a great part of the bandages might with advantage be laid aside particularly the pad and splint that lies upon the wound and that a poultice might probably be substituted with advantage as a detersive.[53]

The management of hernia at the Hôtel-Dieu was also treated at length by Thomson.[54] One case in December 1823 is of particular interest, partly because it offers virtually a complete case-history – only the termination is lacking; and partly because it illuminates the relations between Mortier and the practitioners such as Thomson who attended him. In the course of the operation Mortier pierced the sac with his scalpel; later 'he pointed this out as a fault'. He decided after the hernia had been reduced to pass a thread through the mesentery in order to retain the intestine behind the ring; subsequently he felt the need to 'defend' this decision on the basis of his experience in a previous case. Both these circumstances confirm the impression that Thomson was following a true '*école de perfectionnement*' at which the students themselves possessed a degree of competence that compelled the surgeon to show them a measure of respect; in this context, Mortier was a *primus inter pares* rather than an aloof pedagogue.

The fullest accounts of operative surgery in Thomson's notes do not, however, derive from Mortier's practice, but from that of Janson, the Surgeon-Major of the hospital. Thomson made meticulous reports of two lithotomics performed by Janson in October 1823. The first of these accounts is quoted in full below in order to convey something of the vividness and attention to detail of Thomson's descriptions.

> 16^{nh} 8^{ber} 1823
>
> Saw Mr Janson perform this day the operation for Lithotomy in the recto vesical manner.
>
> The man who is about 30 years of age was mounted on a table on which there was a stuffed cushion covered with leather and over that a wax cloth [here a drawing of this contrivance] an eleve [sic] sat stride legs behind him to support him – his hands and feet were tied in the usual manner and his thighs held apart by assistants – he was placed in a half sit half reclining posture near the edge of the table. A director was introduced into the Urethra which seemed to be somewhat arched in its inferior portion thus [here another drawing]. It was heard very distinctly to strike against the stone – After feeling the catheter thro the rectum with his oiled finger M. J. introduced the scalpel alongside of his left forefinger; taking it in his right [hand] he seemed to push it into the groove of the staff and to cut upwards then taking the staff in his own hand and pulling it towards himself he enlarged the

first wound he made keeping his left forefinger in the bladder he withdrew the knife and staff and introduced the forceps with which after turning them over in the usual french manner two or three times, he seized the stone. On bringing it to the wound it was not without somewhat forcible pulling that he was able to extract it. I did not observe however that any serious laceration of the parts took place and the patient lost very little blood during the operation. The stone was of the mulberry species, very rough upon its surface and round. It was from about 1½ to 1⅔ inch in diameter. A small portion of the surface seemed as if the roughness had been broken down by the forceps. The patient was put to bed without any dressings being applied.

Thomson kept track of this patient for a few days after the operation. His post-operative care devolved upon Mortier. Despite some haemorrhaging he appears to have survived the ordeal.[55]

The second lithotomy, which took place on 30 October, was far more fraught with difficulty; Thomson's disapproval of much that he saw is obvious. He thought that the staff Janson used was 'very clumsily shaped', and considered that, judging by the flow of blood, a false passage had been formed in introducing it. Thomson also doubted whether Janson had indeed struck the stone with the staff. This was a cardinal point as it was an axiom of lithotomy that no operation should be attempted unless the stone was located. Finally, the stone broke in the forceps and had to be extracted in pieces. The patient developed febrile symptoms and died on 1 November.[56]

Various explanations for Thomson's special interest in these operations might be adduced. In the first place, lithotomy occupied a special status for surgeons in the early nineteenth century: it was, in John Bell's words, '*the chef-d'oeuvre* of surgical skill.'[57] Such displays of surgical virtuosity in a foreign hospital were an obvious attraction for any visitor. There was, moreover, a strong family interest in lithotomy. John Thomson had in 1808 published a collection of old papers on the subject to which he appended his own proposals for the improvement of the operation; and two years later produced a pamphlet defending his own skill as a lithotomist.[58] During a visit to Vienna, John Thomson himself, made detailed notes of the mode of lithotomy practised there, although the operations he witnessed were on dead bodies rather than living patients.[59]

In addition, the type of lithotomy William Thomson witnessed in Lyons would have possessed a special interest for him. The recto-vesical method that Janson employed was both innovative and controversial; and this goes far to explain Thomson's attention to operative method, the problems encountered in entering the bladder by this route, and the final outcome of the intervention. Furthermore, Thomson may have had a more specific goal in mind when compiling these observations. Soon after his return to Edinburgh, he applied to become a Fellow of the Royal College of Surgeons. In order to attain this distinction, he was obliged to produce an original dissertation; his chosen topic was lithotomy, with special reference to the recto-vesical operation.

The dissertation contained a number of tables of cases in which this operation had been performed and designed to elucidate the likely results. Most of these, were derived from published sources; but among them were seven lithotomies performed by Janson.[60] The two cases described in the notes can be identified among this group. In the text, Thomson also noted that 'In one of the cases which I saw M. Janson perform the operation, a pair of forceps with broad blades was introduced into the anus, and the gut was dilated transversely by means of them.'[61]

It is impossible to say whether, when he went to Lyons, Thomson had already decided upon the topic of his dissertation for the fellowship and accordingly sought out relevant material, or whether the opportunity to witness Janson's operations suggested the subject to him. But, in either case, these lithotomies illustrate how foreign observations could be made directly serviceable to an individual's career development when he returned home.

The attention to technique in Thomson's account of these operations is consonant with the emphasis upon the practical, manual aspect of surgery evident in the notes. But such concerns did not exhaust the range of Thomson's interests. When he recorded observations of operations for the extirpation of tumours, Thomson complemented his descriptions of the procedures and dressings with a concern for the nature of the growths removed. After an account of a mastectomy performed on 23 September 1823 he noted:

> On being divided the diseased mass seems to exhibit the usual appearance of schirrus (N.B. No central point with diverging laminae). At a number of points, florid red blood seems to have been effused and these points we are disposed to think are softer than the surrounding parts. Quere. Is this the commencement of Fungus Haematodes?[62]

In such passages, Thomson assumes the role of surgeon–pathologist, and in so doing goes beyond the craft concept of surgery. This can be seen as a special case of the clinically orientated pathology discussed above: by combining information gained from a post-operative examination of a tumour with what he knew of the clinical history of the case, he might hope to sharpen his diagnostic and prognostic skills. The above quotation also displays, however, a somewhat more abstract interest in the classification of growths according to current taxonomies. The possibility that a schirrus tumour might metamorphose into fungus haematodes was significant for contemporary debates in pathology. James Wardrop, a familiar of the Thomson family, had in 1809 published an essay arguing that schirrus and fungus haematodes were quite distinct morbid growths.[63]

Just as Carswell's observations hint at the emergence of the 'pure pathologist', so Thomson appears in the manuscript playing the part of the 'scientific surgeon'. Both these roles were still embryonic in form in the 1820s; they were, however, to grow and acquire an imposing stature as the nineteenth century advanced.

These two descriptions – and especially the second – confirm the impression given elsewhere of Thomson as an acute and critical observer of the surgical practice of the Hôtel-Dieu. The attention to technique is also consonant with the emphasis upon the practical, manual aspect of surgery evident in the notes. But while these concerns predominate, they do not exhaust the range of Thomson's interests.

Conclusion

At the outset of this discussion I suggested that Carswell's and Thomson's accounts of their time at the Hôtel-Dieu of Lyons might tell us as much, if not more, about themselves as about what they saw. We have seen how, despite their overt common purpose and a certain amount of common ground, each took a different perspective upon the hospital and made different use of the opportunities that it offered. It has been argued that these divergent points of view correspond to the peculiar interests of two different classes of practitioner: the pure pathologist on the one hand and the scientific surgeon on the other.

It is possible to go a step further. Not only do Carswell's and Thomson's French experiences tell us something about *them*, they are also instructive about *whence they came*. In other words, what these two wrote in Lyons casts light upon contemporary Edinburgh.

This is especially the case with William Thomson's contribution. In the first place, the foci of his attention can be traced to his domestic background and upbringing; in particular, the role of the father in shaping the interests of the son seems to have been major. John Thomson's probable part in sensitizing his son to the issue of surgical appointments, hospital organization, and war wounds has already been noted. The areas of surgical practice – such as hernia and lithotomy – to which William gave special attention also correspond closely to the preoccupations of John Thomson. It is also possible to discern a more general influence. The role of scientific surgeon to which William Thomson aspired was very much defined by John Thomson in his lectures at the Royal College of Surgeons of Edinburgh after 1804. In these lectures, the value of pathological knowledge to the surgeon, rather than mere manual dexterity, was repeatedly stressed.[64]

This emphasis upon the importance of his father in shaping William's orientation as a medical practitioner needs to be qualified by a recognition of the fact that John Thomson was merely one actor – albeit one with exceptional histrionic and stentorian attributes – on the crowded stage of early nineteenth-century Edinburgh medicine. He did not originate the notion of the 'scientific surgeon', although he was crucial in shaping it. The demand for such a concept was, moreover, rooted in the particular circumstances in which Edinburgh surgeons of the period found themselves.

The recognition of this linkage between the nidus of an observer and his perception of an alien context brings with it certain implications. Above all, it underlines Warner's point that the 'transfer' of knowledge from one country to another is a highly involved process. What British students took from France differed significantly from what the Americans derived precisely because each group went with different expectations of the host.[65]

Instead of seeing French medicine as a monolithic structure, the appeal of which can be explained simply by reference to auscultation and the new pathology, France needs to be conceived as a vast medical bazaar with many stalls, each offering a different product. The tastes of the foreign shopper – and therefore what he derived – were shaped above all by his prior experience and future expectations.

We have then to deal, not with a process of passive diffusion but with a true interaction between medical cultures in which the orientation of the visitor was *constitutive* of his perception of and orientation towards a foreign context. The present discussion has, moreover, shown that this interaction cannot be viewed merely at the national level. Particular centres – such as Edinburgh – within Britain generated special types of traveller; while particular institutions in France – such as the Hôtel-Dieu of Lyons – supplied unique opportunities for him to exploit.

Notes

The research on which this paper is based was made possible by the generous support of the Wellcome Trust. I am grateful to the staff of the Special Collections Department of Edinburgh University Library for their assistance. Michael Barfoot, David Hamilton, and John Harley Warner offered valuable comments on an earlier version of the text.

1. Russell C. Maulitz, *Morbid Appearances: The Anatomy of Pathology in the Early Nineteenth Century* (Cambridge, 1987); John Harley Warner, 'The selective transport of medical knowledge: antebellum American physicians and Parisian medical therapeutics', *Bulletin of the History of Medicine*, 59 (1985), 213–31; John Harley Warner, *The Therapeutic Perspective: Medical Practice, Knowledge, and Identity in America, 1820–1885* (Cambridge, Mass., 1986), especially ch. 6.

2. Maulitz, *Morbid Appearances*, pp. 143–6.

3. I have already discussed another portion of this archive in 'Au Lit des Malades: A. F. Chomel's Clinic at the Charité. 1828–29; as reported by Allen Thomson', in W. H. Bynum and Roy Porter (eds), *Brunonianism and Nineteenth-Century European Medicine* (Medical History Supplement, 1988).

4. Carswell Papers, Edinburgh University Library, MS Gen. 590–1; the Lyons notes are in Gen. 591.

5. Gab Despierres, *Histoire de l'Enseignement Médical à Lyon de l'Antiquité à nos Jours* (Lyon, 1984), pp. 80–1; Christian Roche, *L'Enseignement Médical à Lyon de 1821 à 1877: École Secondaire de Médecine (1821–1841) et de Pharmacie (1841–1877)*, Lyons thesis, 1975, p. 13.

6. Ibid., pp. 64–71.

7. See Toby Gelfand, *Professionalizing Modern Medicine: Paris Surgeons and Medical Science and Institutions in the 18th Century* (Westport, 1980), p. 125.

8. On clinical surgical instruction in Edinburgh, see A. Logan Turner, *Story of a Great Hospital: The Royal Infirmary of Edinburgh 1729–1929* (Edinburgh, 1937), pp. 142–6.

9. See the comments on Parisian surgical teaching reported in Othmar Keele, 'La Place et la fonction des modèles étrangers dans la constitution de la problématique hospitalière de l'École de Paris', *History and Philosophy of the Life Sciences*, 6 (1984), 62.

10. Carswell Papers, p. 362.

11. Ibid., p. 357.

12. Ibid.

13. Ibid. A very similar incident was recounted by a French visitor to the Royal Infirmary of Edinburgh in 1827. See L. S. Jacyna, 'The French perception: a medical visitor's view of Scottish medicine in 1827', *Glasgow Medicine*, 6 (November/December 1986), 20.

14. Carswell Papers, p. 358.

15. John Thomson, *Letter to the General Court of Contributors of the Royal Infirmary of Edinburgh; Containing Observations on the Minutes of Evidence, and on the Report of the Committee appointed to enquire into the State of the House. By a Contributor* (Edinburgh, 1818); *A Second Letter to the General Court of Contributors of the Royal Infirmary of Edinburgh; Containing Remarks on the Proceedings at the Meeting held on the 30th March, 1818. To which are annexed, the Report of the Committee* (Edinburgh, 1818).

16. Carswell Papers, p. 358.

17. Ibid., p. 355. The professor's dress was prescribed by law: see Roche, ''Enseignement Médical à Lyon', p. 45.

18. Ibid., p. 360.

19. These controversies are discussed in Michael Barfoot, 'Pedagogy, practice and politics: the Edinburgh medical community in the 18th century', in Malcolm Nicolson (ed.), *Scotland's Health and Medicine* (London, forthcoming).

20. Turner, 1937, *Story of a Great Hospital* p. 372.

21. Carswell Papers, pp. 360, 362. On the functions of the dressers in the Royal Infirmary, see Guenter B. Risse, *Hospital Life in Enlightenment Scotland: Care and Teaching at the Royal Infirmary of Edinburgh* (Cambridge, 1986), pp. 74–5.

22. Carswell Papers, p. 361.

23. See C. J. Lawrence, 'The Edinburgh Medical School and the end of the "old thing" 1790–1830', *History of Universities*, (1988), 259–86.

24. Carswell Papers, p. 327.

25. Ibid., p. 347.
26. Ibid., p. 186.
27. Ibid., p. 295.
28. Ibid., pp. 154–60.
29. Ibid., p. 264.
30. Ibid., p. 209.
31. Ibid.
32. G. N. Cantor, 'The Edinburgh phrenology debates: 1803–1828', *Annals of Science*, 32 (1975), 195–218.
33. Carswell Papers, pp. 232, 265, 273, 277, 341.
34. Ibid., p. 230.
35. Ibid., pp. 163–4.
36. Maulitz, *Morbid Appearances*, p. 135.
37. Carswell Papers, p. 186.
38. Ibid., pp. 218–19.
39. Ibid., pp. 219, 222.
40. Ibid., p. 148.
41. Ibid., p. 169.
42. Ibid., pp. 175–6.
43. Ibid., pp. 208, 227.
44. Ibid., pp. 215, 221.
45. Ibid., pp. 136–7.
46. Ibid., p. 144.
47. Ibid., pp. 259–60.
48. Ibid., pp. 277–8.
49. Ibid., p. 299.
50. Ibid., pp. 269–70.
51. Ibid., pp. 281–2.
52. Ibid., p. 274.
53. Ibid., p. 271.
54. Ibid., pp. 305–14.
55. Ibid., pp. 260–2.
56. Ibid., pp. 255–8.
57. John Bell, *Answer for the Junior Members of the Royal College of Surgeons, of Edinburgh, to the Memorial of Dr James Gregory* (Edinburgh, 1800), p. 20.
58. John Thomson, *Observations on Lithotomy; being a Republication of Dr James Douglas' Appendix to his History of the Lateral Operation for the Stone*, and the other Original Papers relative to Mr Cheselden's Invention and Improvement of that Operation. To which is added, a proposal for a New Manner of Cutting for the stone (Edinburgh, 1808); idem, *Appendix to a Proposal for a new Manner of Cutting for the Stone; Containing an Account of some Cases Operated on after that Manner, in the Royal Infirmary of Edinburgh* (Edinburgh, 1810).
59. John Thomson, [*Journal of his 1814 Visit to France*], National Library of Scotland, MS 9235, pp. 33–4.
60. William Thomson, *A Probationary Essay on the Extraction of Calculi from the Urinary Bladder, containing some Account of certain Methods that have been proposed, submitted by Authority of the President and council, to the Examination of the Royal College of Surgeons of Edinburgh, when a Candidate*

for Admission into their Body, in Conformity to their Regulations respecting the Admission of Ordinary Fellows (Edinburgh, 1825), pp. 44–5, 48.

61. Ibid., p. 13.

62. Ibid., p. 332.

63. James Wardrop, *Observations on Fungus Haematodes or Soft Cancer, in Several of the most Important Organs of the Human Body: Containing also a Comparative View of the Structure of Fungus Haematodes and Cancer. With Cases and Dissections* (Edinburgh, 1809), especially pp. 181–91.

64. A representative part of this course was published: John Thomson, *Lectures on Inflammation, Exhibiting a View of the General Doctrines, Pathological and Practical, of Medical Surgery* (Edinburgh, 1813).

65. Warner, *Therapeutic Perspective*, 1985, esp. p. 214.

6

The idea of science in English medicine: the 'decline of science' and the rhetoric of reform, 1815–45

John Harley Warner

An intensifying preoccupation with the historical relationships among language, meaning, and experience marks what has been called 'the linguistic turn' in recent historiography. Historians have increasingly given serious attention to a view long urged by certain literary critics, sociolinguists, and cultural anthropologists, namely that rhetoric can be regarded less as a vehicle for transmitting information than as a mode of social action that in giving an account of the world imposes a structure and meaning upon it. Language, even language that purports simply to describe, often provides not so much a transcription of life as a model for reordering cultural reality. If language does have such social functions, historians have reasoned, then especially in periods of cultural upheaval one should expect to find particular rhetorical forms that seek both to make sense of a disturbing situation and to articulate a plan by which things can be brought into a more reassuring and satisfying order.[1]

One such rhetorical form – the decline-of-science argument in English medicine – is my focus here. This was the assertion that medical science in England was in relative decline compared with the flourishing state of science in France. Rhetoric about the decline of medical science was partly propelled by the energies that drove the better-known claim that the physical sciences and mathematics in England were in decline; yet the declinist argument in medicine was also firmly rooted in circumstances peculiar to the medical profession. Indeed, by the time Charles Babbage published his *Reflections on the Decline of Science in England* in 1830, the complaint that *medical* science in England was in decline had been audible for more than a decade. Clearly voiced in the 1810s, it became louder in professional rhetoric during the late 1820s and 1830s and persisted into the 1840s.

The decline-of-science argument was one response to the cultural turmoil that so marked the English medical profession between the mid-1810s and the mid-1940s. Those who most energetically used it spoke for general practitioners, a newly self-conscious professional group that held rising aspirations during this period of insecurity and uncertainty. While declinist rhetoric can be interpreted as a straightforward account of the way things were or, again, as a tool contrived by radical reformers to promote professional change, it can also be regarded as one embodiment of deeply held assumptions about the place of science in the intellectual and social order of early and mid-nineteenth-century English medicine. In this chapter I shall analyse the structure and meaning of this rhetoric and, in particular, suggest how it depicted and utilized an idea of science that served both to account for professional disorder and to define and plead for a better way. Reformers found in the language of science a vehicle for comprehending and acting on the sources of disarray in the medical profession. At the same time, in seeking to use science as a professional leaven, they represented a conception of science that was highly specific to their own social and cultural ends.

The 'decline of science' in England and the rise of medicine in France

While the theme of decline in professional rhetoric emerged out of the upheaval of English medical culture, its persistent point of reference was medical ferment on the other side of the Channel. Out of the reorganization of French medicine in the wake of the Revolution – the birth and growth of the clinic that Erwin Ackerknecht and Michel Foucault have described in their very different ways – Paris became a centre unmatched in its medical vitality.[2] French clinicians created fresh models of medical science by exploiting their free access to patients' bodies (living and dead) and new physical and conceptual tools for pathological investigation, such as the stethoscope and physical examination, clinical statistics, and systematic autopsy. For many foreign practitioners the Paris clinic and its products became guides to the cognitive and social transformation of medicine in their own countries.

Medical communication across the Channel had not ceased during the Napoleonic Wars, but after Waterloo English awareness of the medical vigour of Paris mounted sharply. The flow of medical students to the hospitals and dissecting rooms of Paris grew to an exodus during the several decades after 1815.[3] As one wrote home in that year, 'I am tormented by more opportunities than I can embrace.'[4] These travellers returned to England with stories of the Parisian medical world, and were among those who translated French medical writings. The proliferation during this very same period of English medical journals, many of them edited by men uncommonly receptive to French ways, especially drew attention to Parisian activity. Some English medical men even complained that French medicine was being forced upon them by the growing esteem in which it was held by the public (however suspicious the villagers of Middlemarch remained of Tertius Lydgate's Paris credentials). 'My object in coming here', one English medical student wrote from Paris in 1830 to his former preceptor, 'was, that the idea entertained by the world in the present day is that a man can scarcely be able to practice his profession unless he has completed his education in this metropolis; and as I am . . . to be dependent on the opinion of the public and they choose to humble themselves in this way my only course is to sail with the stream.'[5]

With the more ample knowledge of Parisian medicine that came with peace, intensification of comparisons between French and English medicine was virtually inevitable. The English practitioners who visited the newly accessible city in 1815 filled their letters home with not only detailed descriptions of the clinical ideas and methods, institutions, and opportunities for study they found but also their own appraisals of how all these measured up to their London counterparts. Over the next three decades, the letters, diaries, and publications of others who travelled to Paris did the same.[6]

What is especially striking, though, is the singular stridency and sheer durability of one distinct theme about French medicine that emerged in English medical rhetoric. This was the claim that England was behind France in medical *science.* From the mid-1810s through the 1840s, the pivot on which the decline-of-science theme in English medicine turned was an aggressively argued, decidedly invidious comparison of French medical vitality with English medical lethargy: decline did not mean slipping backward, but rather slipping behind France. A London editor writing in the 1830s typically explicated the rapid strides of French science in order to 'expose the truly humiliating, the almost degraded, and the unquestionably backward state of medical science in England'. Taking as his example the most frequently cited paradigm of French medical science, pathology, he noted that 'in France, under a superior system, or one better calculated at least for the *promotion* of science, the disciples of Bichat, and Laennec, have made strides that distance all competitors'. He asserted flatly that 'our continental neighbours have outstripped us beyond dispute – we follow, rather than lead, in the march of medicine'.[7] It was not necessary to say that English medical science was worse off than it had been in earlier decades to claim, as one practitioner did, 'that France in medical science is nearly half a century in advance of England',[8] but only to recognize French achievement. The exodus of Englishmen to Paris for medical study, the growing reliance on French medical literature, and the prominent proselytism of some English converts to French medical ways all made French ascendancy in medical science increasingly blatant if not unmistakable.

Degradation proclaimed: science and the general practitioner

The robustness of the Paris clinic did pose in some ways a disturbing contrast to English torpor. But however solid the evidential foundation for this argument may have been, it does not explain why many English medical practitioners chose to publicly draw attention to this humiliating state of affairs – why, that is, they elected to celebrate national inferiority (especially to France) rather than to gloss over it. Often the tone in which the declinist argument was voiced was not grudging, doleful, or sulky, but brash, urgent, and even proselytizing. What needs to be explained is not so much the content of the claim that English medical science was inferior, but the vigour with which many medical men proclaimed that perception.[9]

One kind of explanation is suggested by historians' interpretations of other decline-of-science claims – claims about the physical sciences in Italy in the 1910s, the sciences at large in France in the 1860s, the medical sciences in the American South in the 1850s, and Babbage's claims about the physical sciences and mathematics in England in the 1830s.[10] As with all of these, I want to suggest that the *stridency* of complaints about the decline of medical science in England came primarily from reformist energies. Statements about English backwardness were usually framed in the context of explanations for French achievements. And it was at this point that the link connecting the decline argument with programmes for reform was welded. Declinist claims usually were made in order to set up the question, What is holding English medical science back? In the appraisal of reformers, the rise of French medical science demonstrated the superiority of the system of medical polity from which that science emerged. Invidious comparisons ordinarily urged changes in English medical polity modelled selectively on the French example. The energetic declaration that England was woefully behind France in medical science functioned as a professional jeremiad: it was a lamenting and denunciatory complaint about things as they were, but more, it was also a call for repentance that spelled out what needed to be done in order to attain professional salvation.

Comparisons that found English medical science wanting were not confined to any single group among English practitioners. Nevertheless, it is possible to identify the distinguishing orientations of those who made the most of England's putative backwardness and those who made the least of it.[11] By and large, those who most noticeably dismissed or muffled grumblings about decline belonged to the socially and institutionally entrenched élite, the leaders of the corporations and physicians and surgeons to the metropolitan hospitals. Sometimes they condemned excessive zeal for French science, what one called 'the absurd Frenchified system now vigorously attempted to be palmed upon them' and what another stigmatized as the pathological behaviour of those he diagnosed as 'Gallomaniacs'.[12] They also denounced the radicalism of medical men who recklessly sacrificed English honour by upholding medical models of what one critic called 'French reform – or rather revolution'. 'Our *ultra*-reformers,' he continued, 'look across the straits of Dover whenever they want something to put in the place of what displeases them at home.'[13]

But the established élite tended not to dwell on the state of English *science*, and elected instead to concentrate on the excellencies of English *practice*. This valuation of practice above all else, they asserted, properly informed the intellectual and institutional structure of English medicine. 'It is one advantage arising from the peculiar constitution of the London medical schools, that, with few exceptions, the instructions, which you here receive, have in a greater or lesser degree, *a tendency to practice*,' Sir Benjamin C. Brodie, Bart., FRS, told his students in 1838.

> The ambition of the teacher of Anatomy is not limited to success in his present vocation. He looks forward to the time when his profession as a Physician or Surgeon will elevate him to fame and fortune. . . . I have no doubt that the praises which are bestowed on some of the continental anatomists are well founded: that there are universities in which the anatomical professors, devoting their whole time, and industry, and intellect, to this one pursuit, explain the mysteries of minute anatomy at greater length, and with more precision, than the teachers here: but nevertheless, I assert that ours is the better method with a view to the education of those who wish to become *not mere philosophers, but skilful and useful practitioners.*[14]

The decline-of-science argument in medicine, unlike the one in the physical sciences and mathematics, was less a controversy than a persistent theme, and those who would defend English medicine generally avoided the open confrontation that efforts to systematically disprove claims of French superiority in science would incite.

On the other hand, those who made the most of the decline argument were among those most anxious for change. But they were not all cast in a single mould. A small number of them were engaged in scientific activity along Parisian lines, and used the decline argument to bolster support for their own scientific programmes. Other reformers who used the decline argument were provincial medical entrepreneurs seeking a redistribution of professional power between metropolis and province. Some ambitious provincial practitioners – especially those involved in building institutions such as infirmaries, societies, and schools –

used declinism as a weapon in assailing London's hegemony in medicine and what they depicted as the consequent depression of English medical science. By using the decline argument they hoped to elevate provincial medical enterprise and with it their own position.[15]

But while various reform interests pressed the decline argument into their service, overwhelmingly the most strident declinists saw themselves as champions of the cause of general practitioners. The decline argument as they used it, the focus here, both explained a disturbing situation and made the case for reforms, patterned very selectively on the Parisian model, that would give the general practitioner recognition, status, and institutional support, and at the same time establish his professional legitimacy. Ardent declinism correlated well with a declared dedication to general practitioners' interests. As medical periodicals grew more strident in their advocacy of reform for the general practitioners, for example, their use of the decline argument in turn grew louder and more frequent. In the 1820s the *Lancet* was probably the most vital forum of radical declinism, but by the early 1840s its position had been supplanted by the *Medical Times.* At the same time, the latter journal had vigorously taken up the cause of general practitioners. 'The Lancet is now more decent & less tricky than formerly – but ye Medical Times is the most scurrilous abusive lying & villainous that ever disgraced our Literature,' one surgeon complained to a colleague in 1846.

> It is running the course the Lancet did to raise its circulation & finds out that abusing whatever is respectable, & flattering the Genl Practers (by which last is meant just the lowest grade, & necessarily the most numerous of the (regular) Profession & not an Individual Member of the Profn who stands high as a Genl Practr) is the way to obtain its selfish Object.[16]

The emergence of a collective self-consciousness among English general practitioners, their growing sense of corporate identity and aspirations for uplift during precisely the period when awareness of French vitality was mounting, and when the decline argument emerged and came to thrive, has been clearly mapped by Irvine Loudon and others. They have shown that although those known as apothecaries, surgeon-apothecaries, or increasingly as general practitioners made up the vast majority of the profession, they stood at its margins in status and legitimacy. The very scope of general practitioners' practice separated them from 'pure' physicians and surgeons, a symbolic distinction in role that reflected a more profound distinction in social accomplishment and status. The élite practitioner's prestige came principally not from the practice of his vocation or mastery of medical knowledge but from his social origins, family connections, and gentlemanly achievement. As long as professional status was tied to an artificial separation in principle between the branches of medicine, general practitioners were consigned to a degraded position. And because most practitioners could not reasonably aspire to the trappings of gentility and access to patronage that conferred status on the élite, they had only limited prospects for upward mobility. Individually, the justification for claims to distinction they might make, of medical knowledge and skill, was of limited utility. Collectively, their inability to raise educational and licensing standards without support from the Colleges and their bondage to trade through the Society of Apothecaries blocked efforts to improve the group's standing.[17] It was this situation that reformers sought both to explain and to reorder by energetically deploying the decline-of-science argument.

Declinism and reform

Declinist rhetoric used to urge reform conformed to a strikingly persistent pattern, which can be displayed by giving, if only schematically, the place of the decline argument in three examples broadly familiar to historians. Through the early 1830s, one of the most touted restraints on English medical science was the dearth of corpses available for anatomical teaching and investigation. A legal system that compelled anatomists to rely on the illegal traffic of the body-snatcher stigmatized all who anatomized and raised the cost of extensive study beyond many students' means. This depressed the level of knowledge about normal and pathological anatomy among English practitioners and hampered new contributions.

The abundant, cheap, legal supply of bodies that was a major draw to Paris was a standing backdrop for denunciations of the English system. It went far towards explaining French achievements and what one observer referred to as 'the immense number of medical students . . . daily flocking to Paris'.[18] 'The obstacles which impede the study of anatomy in this country are such, and the facilities presented to the study in foreign countries are so great, that those English students who are desirous of obtaining a thorough knowledge of the science desert the schools at home, and repair to those abroad,' the Committee of the House of Commons appointed to investigate the difficulties of anatomizing in England reported in 1828. 'Their principal resort is to Paris, where 200 English students of anatomy are now pursuing their course of instruction.' Thus, in testimony before the Parliamentary Committee, witnesses persistently urged legislation modelled after the French plan to provide anatomical material. 'They dwell upon the practice of the schools of Paris,' a writer in the *London Medical and Physical Journal* explained, 'because it approaches most nearly to the plan recommended by most of the witnesses for adoption in this country.'[19] English laws suppressed anatomy, most who testified agreed, and change depended on the Government. What was needed, reformers insisted, was legislation modelled after the French plan to provide anatomical material.[20]

A second source of the depressed condition of medical science was the misgovernment of London's hospitals. According to declinist writings, private control of these institutions by men who did not particularly care about science meant that England's richest resource for generating and disseminating medical knowledge was underexploited. Critics charged that nepotism, social influence, and commercial connections, not skill or scientific ability, figured most prominently in appointments of medical officers. 'There is scarcely a physician or surgeon attached, to an hospital or dispensary in London, who has not obtained his appointment through interest, vote-making, or intrigue, and not one on the grounds of knowledge, experience, or eminence,' one observer commented in 1833.[21] Those who possessed the opportunities for clinical research did not necessarily have the interest or aptitude for pursuing it, while practitioners more committed to the production of new knowledge were denied access to patients. Further, hospital physicians and surgeons regarded teaching more as a means of making money than as an obligation of their office, and the stiff fees they charged for hospital teaching barred many students from access to scientific knowledge. 'I am completely sick of this system of extortion, of taxes upon knowledge,' one pupil at a London hospital in 1834 wrote to his mother. 'This plan is full of corruption.'[22] As with the supply of dead bodies, so too the access to living ones was stymied by English medical polity.

France, again, was a comparison by which English hospital government was judged to retard science. As declinist Michael Ryan put it, 'While the French physician is pursuing science, the English physician is hunting fees.'[23] In Paris, critics of the London hospitals maintained, not patronage but scientific merit determined clinical appointments. Such a system tended to favour clinicians dedicated to research, and gave them a state salary that severed their income from student fees. Further, the French student, unlike his English counterpart, gained access to the hospitals by ability in medicine rather than ability to pay. 'In England, no appointments are obtained from merit alone, but by the base and dishonest means of private, monied, family, or clique interest,' one English practitioner wrote from Paris. 'In England, where money is the test of respectability and professional talent, they *purchase* their appointments by the twelvemonth,' he continued. 'In France the desideratum which the system espouses is talent – talent making the way to preferment; in England it is money and family patronage.'[24] Accordingly, some reformers urged that legislated reconstruction of hospital management, patterned after the Paris mode of placing patient care, teaching, and research under state control, would lead to science's rebirth in the English clinic.

A third cause of England's backwardness was the low esteem accorded to science by the profession's institutional leaders, those whom declinist Thomas Wakley called 'mercenary, goose-brained monopolists and charlatans'.[25] Reformers assailed the Royal Colleges of Physicians and Surgeons for favouring social over scientific qualifications, thereby devaluing science as a determinant of professional recognition and smothering incentive to scientific enterprise. 'The old corporations,' one practitioner noted, 'are obsolete – effete – moribund. They form in their cadaverous aspect the vivid contrast to the life and freshness of science that is on the wing abroad.'[26] Looking at the leadership of the corporations, 'the characteristic which stands out most prominently is certainly not its science,' another critic commented in 1843. 'Our chiefs,' he continued, 'are recipients of so much per annum (their *private* property being the most valued item) – they are denizens of an aristocratic square –

acquaintances of the noble – agreeable fellows in society – carriage-owners – gentlemen – – bustling men of business; any thing, in short, but those patronized humble beings – *men of science.*'[27] More than this, because the Apothecaries' Hall and Surgeons' College functioned as *de facto* licensing bodies, they were in a position to regulate scientific standards in education. Yet, for example, the records of the Society of Apothecaries make it clear that at least through the 1830s deficiency in Latin, not in science, was the most common reason some candidates for the licence were failed.[28] By keeping formal requirements and knowledge actually tested in examinations low, the established élites depressed the scientific education of English practitioners.

This situation was turned on its head in France, reformers maintained, where medical government sustained the prestige of science and encouraged its pursuit by making scientific achievement the cardinal claim to professional reward. Therefore, giving scientific accomplishment an importance in assigning professional rank comparable to what reformers believed it had in France and making requirements for qualifications more rigorous were pivotal in plans for invigorating English medical science. If the Colleges would not take up this change of their own accord, then it should be imposed upon them by legislation.[29]

These examples could be greatly multiplied and greatly refined. But what is clear enough in these instances and evident in others as well is that by the 1820s the decline-of-science argument had become part of an almost standardized rhetorical formula that could be placed in aid of a wide array of professional reforms. It was one part of a larger argument that conformed to a fixed pattern, though often an author presented only portions of it. Typically, the writer asserted that medical science in England was in decline, identified a source of its low standing, and explicated how it kept science down. He next turned to the comparable situation on the Continent, usually France, and showed how the French system better nurtured science. Having established the need for change and pointed to the appropriate model (and usually having affirmed the importance of science to the medical profession), he then proposed how change after a French blueprint could elevate medical science in England. The argument was often closed with a codicil, which stated that ultimately the reforms declinists sought required legislative intervention.

I want to emphasize that declinist rhetoric fixed squarely upon *science*; this was not an argument about the decline of English medicine at large. Even those who most energetically extolled French superiority in medical science maintained that, as one English declinist modestly put it, 'We are indisputably the best practitioners in the world.'[30] Arguing that English practitioners were 'outstripped in the pursuit of scientific medicine by our brethren of France', one writer in 1835 typically qualified his remarks by adding,

> We do not mean to say that British practitioners are inferior in their treatment of disease; on the contrary, we believe that they have, in this respect, greatly the advantage of those of any other nation; but we do say with regret, that more is at present doing toward enlargening the boundaries of the science on the continent than in England.[31]

'The French took the lead in pathological anatomy,' another practitioner observed, 'the English in practical utility – in the power of mitigating human suffering, and saving life.'[32]

French clinicians were stereotyped as ardent in their desire to understand disease but apathetic in their efforts to cure it. 'I thought the French students more curious to know precisely the situation of the disease than interested in its treatment,' one practitioner visiting Paris in 1828 typically wrote home. 'Indeed, they seem to think that the perfection of medicine consists not so much in keeping patients alive as in foretelling with precision the appearances which will be found after death.'[33] Oftentimes praise for French science was followed by explicit parenthetical cautions against its practice. 'It is remarkable that, with all the light to be derived from morbid anatomy, the treatment of disease should be so deplorably bad in that country,' one English practitioner wrote.[34] By contrast, the English portrayed themselves as pre-eminently practical. Thus, the same reformers who asserted the superiority of French science routinely insisted on the superiority of English practice.

Science and professional order

It was the complaint that French medical *science* had surpassed that of England, then, that became a common convention for criticizing the prevailing order and demanding change after a French model. 'It is the science-killing tendencies of our old corporations that have awakened in us the whole severity of our opposition to them,' one declinist asserted in lambasting the Colleges and Hall for keeping educational standards low. Seconding the condemnation of the corporations by the National Association of General Practitioners, he charged, 'All our statements resolve themselves ultimately into the one grand accusation – they oppose the progress of science.'[35] In declinist polemics, the élite's neglect of science and neglect of the general practitioner, leading to the degradation of both, were often coupled. In 1836 George Webster told the organizing meeting of the first British Medical Association, assertively a society of general practitioners,

> Had the constituted authorities done their duty . . . we should not have been obliged to meet this night, to take the matter into our own hands, and form an association. But instead of protecting the *profession*, I fear they have frequently oppressed it; in the place of advancing *science*, I fear they have rather acted as drags on the wheels of improvement.[36]

In reform programmes, on the other hand, science and the general practitioner would be elevated together. Giving students freer access to hospital wards as in Parisian institutions, for example, or increasing the scientific knowledge required for qualification, would uplift the profession's standards and scientific acumen. The connection between science and the corporate aspirations of general practitioners was made tightly in some of the earliest clear demands to put general practitioners on an equal footing with physicians and surgeons. In writing to a legislative patron on 'the present condition of the medical profession', as early as 1813, Edward Barlow, prominent as an early activist, argued that the established corporations'

> existence has tended more to retard than accelerate the progress of that art over which they presided, – and that

> this if left to the influence of popular sentiment alone, would have acquired a much higher degree of perfection, whether we regard its [that is, the medical profession's] interests as a Science, – or its establishment as a political institution, considerations by the by more intimately connected than is generally imagined, – than it has now attained.[37]

Yet, in using the decline argument, these reformers were looking for more than institutional change. They also claimed for science a fundamentally new importance to the English medical profession. Certainly the early-nineteenth-century physician or surgeon regarded natural science as one part of his domain, but it was not what principally set him apart from lower orders of practitioners. Declinist writings, on the contrary, conventionally placed science at the heart of professional identity. Thus, in assailing the medical élite for neglecting science, one reformer typically affirmed that 'the real distinction, the true respectability of our profession, is its science. It is to us what valour is to the soldier, piety to the priest, chastity to woman. . . . It is our only title to existence as a profession – our only claim to support.'[38]

It was in part the chasm separating this image of science as the most powerful symbol of professional identity from the reality of professional definition derived from social position that seemed to reformers to give the idea of science such promise as a tool in promoting professional change. Just as reformers set up organizations for general practitioners outside existing professional structures, and looked across the Channel for medical models to emulate, so too they sought to establish an alternative professional value system in which claims to status and legitimacy would be based upon an allegiance to science. Practitioners who could not reasonably aspire to the gentlemanly manner of living and social patronage on which advancement chiefly depended could, in principle, excel sufficiently in science to claim some measure of elevation. As important, grounding professional identity on scientific knowledge meant that raising scientific standards for general practitioners could improve their status as a group, and in the process distance them from the dispensing druggists and irregular practitioners who threatened competition from below.

Unable to advance the profession as a whole from within the established system, reformers went outside it to find in science the distinctive nucleus for a new ideology of professional identity. Dissenting from the sources of professional distinction that prevailed in the Royal Colleges, they urged that 'there is another and far more influential tribunal to which they may appeal, in support of the honour and dignity of their profession – that of science. Let knowledge and learning, and those only, be the passport to their Halls.' A new kind of college, possessing 'a far higher name in science, and a far greater moral influence in the state, than it does at present', should be established 'with knowledge and experience, not place and privilege, as the passport to its honours'.[39] In support of their demand that science become the new arbiter of professional place and prestige, declinists endlessly cited the supposed meritocracy of French medicine. Practitioners and students should, for example, obtain hospital appointments as they did in France, by *concours* or public competitions that displayed and tested their knowledge. Similarly, the Colleges should judge scientific and medical acquirements more than social ones in selecting whom they would elevate.[40]

Reformers further invoked the interests of science and the French example as their authority in calling for a unified profession. Their demands for uniform education, examination, licensing, and registration of all medical practitioners represented in part a desire to improve scientific standards. At the same time, such measures were designed to erode the distinctions that kept the *general* practitioner on the margins of professional legitimacy. They were a protest against 'the distinction of ranks in what ought to be the commonwealth of science'.[41] Science, reformers argued, made no distinction between physic and surgery. Their traditional separateness should therefore be abolished, and the profession reconstituted with general practice as its model and science as its justification. Reformers looked forward to a time when 'the WHOLE PROFESSION will be recognised as *one body*, enjoying equal rights and privileges – in which talent will be honoured, and industry rewarded, and where distinctions in rank can only coexist with distinctions in merit'.[42] The general practitioner would be set up as the norm in a unified profession encompassing all branches of medicine. In the new ideology of professional identity, 'pure' physicians and surgeons had no sanction for their specialized role, and if they persisted in it would be the ones on the margins. Tellingly, declinist rhetoric often redefined 'the medical profession' as a body of general practitioners to which 'pure' physicians and surgeons were, as one reformer put it, 'offsets' and 'parasites'.[43]

The use of scientific culture by English medical practitioners to increase status and enhance identity was not of course novel. Some élite surgeons, for example, as Stephen Jacyna has pointed out, had sought to elevate their prestige by identification with a learned tradition science represented.[44] Scientific surgery, self-consciously traced back to Hunter, offered a platform for group professional uplift. 'There was a time when surgeons were considered as mere appendages to physicians[,] the mere operators who were to be put in motion by their directions,' a surgical pupil attending John Abernethy's lectures in 1812 wrote in his class notebook. 'But times are changing & surgeons have changed too – They have been hard working men – have studied ye animal economy – & in consequence have got a kind of information wch. puts them above this tuition (I might say) – at least puts them upon a par wth. others of yr. profession.'[45] The rhetoric of science may actually have become less appealing to these surgeons as spokesmen for the general practitioners came to cast their reform language partly in the idiom of 'radical science'.

Still, the *kinds* of changes those speaking for general practitioners called for in the name of science were singularly thoroughgoing. They sought the prestige that conspicuous possession of scientific culture could confer; but, more than this, they used science as a platform from which to demand fundamental changes patterned after a selectively constructed model of French medical polity – that is, the French profession's social and legal organization, rewards system, relationship with the state, and institutional arrangements.

These reformers produced rhetoric about the decline of science for several audiences. They saw themselves speaking primarily to the masses of the profession, the general practitioners whose collective position they hoped to elevate. Through the decline argument, they explained to the rank and file the causes of their degradation and identified those to blame. Further, by showing general practitioners the possibility of upward mobility, reformers sought to mobilize them into an energetic and vocal body standing united under the banner of science.

Reformers were speaking as well to a broader lay audience, especially those in a position to legislate change, and did so in language designed to tap into the power of English chauvinism to motivate action. They were self-consciously playing on what one French surgeon described as 'the national pride of the English, which is greater, perhaps, that that of any other civilized nation'.[46] Stridently asserting the superiority of the French in medical science would 'stimulate the apathy of the members of our Legislature by frequently holding before their eyes the example of other nations'.[47] And, at least implicitly, the appeal to nationalistic pride by a display of French cultural achievement also urged the established medical élite to recognize and accept its responsibility for upholding science and the profession.

Above all, though, these reformers were speaking to each other and to themselves. Through their oratory they made professional degradation understandable and affirmed that they knew the solution. Their production of rhetoric was itself one form of action; aside from exhibiting their leadership, it may have provided the reassuring sense of doing something to promote professional redemption. It also gave reformers the satisfaction of denouncing high-placed sinners and exhorting them to repent while at the same time declaring as evidence of their own sanctity their allegiance to science.[48]

A comparative perspective on the meaning of science

As the historiography of the past decade has stressed, however, the idea of science in medicine was extraordinarily malleable, frequently holding divergent meanings for different people and nearly always conveying multiple connotations simultaneously.[49] Just what was it that these reformers spoke of when they used the term *science*? Certainly many contributors to the declinist rhetoric held quite specific and well-elaborated notions of what constituted science. For example, among the activists in the first British Medical Association, which from its founding in 1836 was one forum for strident declinist rhetoric, were such men as William Farr, Robert Grant, Augustus Bozzi Granville,

Marshall Hall, James Johnson, Robert Liston, and Thomas Wakley. Yet, even though some of them were highly reflective about the substance of natural scientific knowledge as well as its imagery, in using this language of professional reform that they shared in common they frequently spoke of science without pointing to any particular method or body of know- ledge.[50] Often the declinists' comparisons of England with France referred to the concrete content of medical science – knowledge about pathological anatomy, for instance; but such discrete comparisons, as I have suggested, informed a broader argument about the place of *science* in the English medical profession in which the meaning of that term was much more problematic.

To clarify this idea of science, I want to compare the decline-of-science rhetoric with another contemporaneous and equally vigorous argument for professional reform that also took the superiority of French medical science as its premise. This was a theme used by medical reformers in the United States. I will sketch this American rhetoric very briefly, then use it as a device to sharpen those features that English reformers most commonly and boldly expressed in their representations of science.[51]

During the first half of the nineteenth century, in the United States as in England there was a widespread perception that the regular medical profession was degraded. And among the most energetic reformers were those who, like the English declinists, maintained that the example of superior French science offered a guide to professional and social uplift. What some Americans perceived as so promising in French medical science was its characteristic epistemological stance, a denunciation of rationalism and commitment to sensual empiricism. French medical science surpassed that of all other countries, these American reformers argued, and the chief reason was the epistemology that was its most notable feature. The degradation of the orthodox profession – epitomized by the strength of such competing sectarians as botanic practitioners and homeopathists – was largely explained by a misguided allegiance to rationalism. If, however, Americans would but take up the epistemology responsible for French success in *science*, the argument continued, then they (being practical Americans) could attain comparable success in transforming medical *practice*. Greater success in practice in turn would let orthodox practitioners edge out those most blameful for holding down the profession, their sectarian competitors, and would improve the position of the regular medical profession in American society.[52]

Without elaborating on the complexities of the American case, it should none the less be clear that, both in England and in the United States, some reformers made French medical science the centrepiece of vigorous and durable arguments for reform. In both rhetorical themes, the superiority of French medical science was the premise. In both again, the account given for why French science was superior also explained the relative inferiority of English or American science and the degradation of the profession. And, in both, certain characteristic features of French science were held up as guides to change and, thereby, professional uplift. Finally, in both, a proclaimed allegiance to science was in the final analysis the justification for denouncing the established order and calling for specific changes. However, the depictions of science that American and English reformers presented differed in quite significant ways; and the contrast accentuates the most prominent attributes of 'science' as the English declinists represented it.[53]

To begin with, in the American reform rhetoric, science was quite commonly depicted as a force for change in practice. It was in its power to transform behaviour at the bedside that the promise of science to improve the lot of the medical profession ultimately rested. By contrast, the idea of science presented in declinist rhetoric made relatively little reference to its power to alter practice. English reformers were convinced, after all, that in their country ability in medicine had by comparison little to do with professional status.

What Americans had in mind in envisioning science as a tool in reconstructing practice was science not as a particular body of knowledge but as a particular epistemological stance, and this was another feature of science they highlighted. American reformers endlessly belaboured the point that science meant empiricism. Parisian clinical empiricism would improve regular performance in an open medical market-place, with public approbation conferring prestige in a society committed to egalitarianism. But for English reformers speaking for general practitioners, whether empiricism was a potent device in changing medical knowledge was not really the issue; as an instrument in professional change, it appeared less likely to work well within the English system than within the American one, and no particular epistemology was prominently identified with the idea of science portrayed in declinist writings.

In English rhetoric, science often stood for the system of medical polity that supported or oppressed it, but this was not common in the language of American reformers. In speaking of French science, for example, the Americans only seldom presented it as a vehicle for ushering in features of French medical polity, such as rigorous educational and licensing standards. The political power of populism at this time was leading to the abolition of medical licensing laws across the United States, and a campaign to elevate professional standards by legislative enactment seemed to many plainly bootless. But, for English reformers, presenting the superiority of French science as above all testimony to the nurturing policies of the French state was key. Part of what they wanted was more rigorous scientific standards for qualification. English reformers commonly depicted science as a sensitive gauge to the vigour or frailty of the system of medical polity from which it emerged.

Further, in the American reform language there was virtually no depiction whatsoever of science as an emblem of meritocracy. Science, that is, was not envisaged as a club useful in beating down special privilege and thereby advancing the profession. This is not to deny the importance of social connections or nepotism in American medicine or the fact that regular practitioners pointed to their allegiance to science as one of the traits that made them superior to other practitioners. But in American society, wherein *all* claims to special privilege were under popular siege, regular medical practitioners were unlikely to accentuate an image of science calculated to urge further democratization. As should be clear, though, in the English decline argument meritocracy was an ideal deeply embedded in the portrayal of science.

Finally, the English reformers tended to portray science as an intrinsically desirable commodity that they expected to confer prestige upon its possessors, but this was an expectation far from self-evident among the Americans. In the United Stages during this period, where claims to status based on special learning were under attack and the professions especially beset, science offered medical practitioners a doubtfully reliable source of cultural accreditation. By contrast, English reformers represented an infusion of scientific culture into the medical rank and file as a promising way to raise up the profession as a body. So, too, they depicted science as a suitable core for the general practitioner's professional identity, whereas before the final third of the century American medical men spoke of science as only one component in professional identity, one that was corrupting if taken up in the extreme and at all events subordinate to the chief source of professional definition, which was practice.

The idea of science

My aim in contrasting these two languages of professional reform, both of which took a proclaimed admiration for French medical science as their core, has been to help sharpen some of the most vivid and most characteristic features of the idea of science deployed in the English decline-of-science rhetoric. The science that English reformers depicted, unlike that of their American counterparts, did not in any large measure derive its importance from its promise to transform medical practice. Nor was it an image of science that necessarily featured any body of medical knowledge in particular or, again unlike the American depiction, any particular epistemology. It was, however, an image that tended to identify science with professional polity, that is the principles ruling professional organization, the conferral of status and definition of identity, the relationship between the profession and the state, and criteria for distributing professional rewards, as well as the value system that undergirded all of these.

Not just the use reformers made of the idea of science, but also the very idea of science they chose to represent was neatly fitted to the specific problems and possibilities of their own culture. In the decline-of-science argument, English medical reformers drew selectively on French examples to urge the reforms in medical polity that they sought. At the same time, they portrayed a conception of science that was quite specific to the perceived needs of general practitioners as a group within English society, a conception of science calculated to bring order to their professional world. The meanings vested in science, in other words, were fundamentally shaped by the peculiar circumstances and aspirations of the men who made it so prominent in their rhetoric, shaped not just by the broader values of English or medical culture at large but also by the specific purposes the language was designed to serve. The medical practitioner who suggested the analogy in the mid-nineteenth century might not have approved of putting it this way, but *science*, both as an idea and as a polemical device used to direct behaviour, was in some respects very much indeed like valour, piety, and chastity.[54]

Notes

For their comments on much earlier versions of this essay, I am grateful to William Coleman, Frederic L. Holmes, Christopher Lawrence, and M. Jeanne Peterson. This paper was supported in part by a research fellowship from the Wellcome Trust.

1. I draw heavily here on Drew Gilpin Faust, 'The rhetoric and ritual of agriculture in antebellum South Carolina', *Journal of Southern History*, 45 (1979), 303–28. William J. Bowsma discusses 'the linguistic turn' in 'Intellectual history in the 1980s: from history of ideas to history of meaning', *Journal of Interdisciplinary History*, 12 (1981), 279–91, p. 290; and see Martin Jay, 'Should intellectual history take a linguistic turn? reflections on the Habermas-Gadamer debate', in Dominick LaCapra and Steven L. Kaplan (eds), *Modern European Intellectual History: Reappraisals and New Perspectives* (Ithaca and London: Cornell University Press, 1982), pp. 86–110, and John E. Toews, 'Intellectual history after the linguistic turn: the autonomy of meaning and the irreducibility of experience', *American Historical Review*, 92 (1987), 879–907.

2. Erwin H. Ackerknecht, *Medicine at the Paris Hospital, 1794–1848* (Baltimore and London: Johns Hopkins University Press, 1967); Michel Foucault, *The Birth of the Clinic: An Archaeology of Medical Perception*, trans. A. M. Sheridan Smith (New York: Pantheon Books, 1973 [Paris, 1963]).

3. On the migration of English students to Paris, see Pierre Huard and Mirko D. Grmek, 'Les élèves étranges de Laennec', *Revue d'histoire des sciences*, 26 (1973), 315–37; Russell C. Maulitz, 'Channel crossing: the lure of French pathology for English medical students, 1816–36', *Bulletin of the History of Medicine*, 55 (1981), 475–96; and Russell C. Maulitz, *Morbid Appearances: The Anatomy of Pathology in the Early Nineteenth Century* (Cambridge: Cambridge University Press, 1987). Typical indicators of French ascendancy are 'Causes of the slow advancement of medical science', *Lancet*, 2 (1837–8), 778–82, p. 779; Charles Higgins, *Observations on Climate, Diet and Medical Treatment in France and England* (London: Burgess & Hill, 1835), pp. 86–7; 'Introductory lecture, &c.', *Transactions of the Associated Apothecaries and Surgeon-Apothecaries of England and Wales*, 1 (1823), iii–cxxxviii, p. xciv;

J. F. South, 'Lectures on natural and morbid anatomy and physiology delivered by John Abernethy Esq FRS in the anatomical theatre at St Bartholomew's Hospital in the years 1819 & 1820, vol. 1, lecture of 2 October [1819]', Library, Royal College of Surgeons, London; and Silas Stedman, Lectures on the materia medica [given by] Dr Chomeley at Guys Hospital, 1817, Library, Royal College of Physicians, London.

4. John Green Crosse, 'Lettre 19eme', in, Letters from Paris, 1814–1815, 2 vols. (MS 473–474), in John Green Crosse Papers, Norfolk Record Office, Central Library, Norwich, vol. 2, p. 115.

5. Benjamin Phillips to Henry Daniel, Paris, 29 May 1830, Bristol Infirmary Biographical Memoirs, vol. 10 (1825–30), Bristol Record Office, The Council House, Bristol, p. 22.

6. For medical comparisons of the newly opened city of Paris with London, see Crosse, Letters from Paris, 1814–1815, Crosse Papers; James Haddy James to Benjamin Fuller, Esqr., Paris, 18 October 1815, James Haddy James Papers, Devon Record Office, Exeter; and James Haddy James, Diary, Paris, 1815, in James Papers.

7. 'State of medical science in England', *London Medical Gazette*, 7 (1830–1), 274–8, pp. 275, 278.

8. 'The French hospitals and medical schools', *Medical Times*, 1 (1839–40), 2–4, p. 4.

9. I am not concerned here with assessing the actual balance between English and French medical accomplishment, though I would say that the relatively greater vigour of French medical science as a whole is easy to see if tedious to show. If the opposite were the case, however, and English science superior to French, it would point all the more strongly to the fact that the decline-of-science claim in medicine was much more than a simple description of things as they were.

10. The large literature that touches upon the decline-of-science controversy in which Babbage was the most prominent player includes Susan Faye Cannon, *Science in Culture: The Early Victorian Period* (New York: Dawson and Science History Publications, 1978); George A. Foote, 'The place of science in the British Reform Movement 1830–1850', *Isis*, 42 (1951), 192–208; Marie Boas Hall, *All Scientists Now: The Royal Society in the Nineteenth Century* (Cambridge: Cambridge University Press, 1984); J. B. Morrell, 'Individualism and the structure of British science in 1830', *Historical Studies in the Physical Sciences*, 3 (1971), 183–204; J. B. Morrell and Arnold Thackray, *Gentlemen of Science: Early Years of the British Association for the Advancement of Science* (Oxford: Clarendon Press, 1981); A. D. Orange, 'The British Association for the Advancement of Science: the provincial background', *Science Studies*, 1 (1971), 315–39; A. D. Orange, 'The origins of the British Association for the Advancement of Science', *British Journal for the History of Science*, 6 (1972), 152–76; Nathan Reingold, 'Babbage and Moll on the state of science in Great Britain: a note on a document', *British Journal for the History of Science*, 4 (1968), 58–64; and L. Pearce Williams, 'The Royal Society and the founding of the British Association for the Advancement of Science', *Notes and Records of the Royal Society*, 16 (1961), 221–33. On other decline-of-science controversies,

see Rainald von Gizycki, 'Centre and periphery in the international scientific community: Germany, France and Great Britain in the 19th century', *Minerva*, 11 (1973), 474–94; Mary Jo Nye, 'Scientific decline: is quantitative evaluation enough?' *Isis*, 75 (1984), 697–708; Barbara J. Reeves, 'Money, status, jobs, and lobbies: the social functions of decline of science claims', paper presented at the History of Science Society annual meeting, Philadelphia, 30 October 1982; and John Harley Warner, 'The idea of Southern medical distinctiveness: medical knowledge and practice in the Old South', in Judith Walzer Leavitt and Ronald L. Numbers (eds), *Sickness and Health in America: Readings in the History of Medicine and Public Health*, 2nd edn (Madison and London: University of Wisconsin Press, 1985), pp. 53–70 (and, for the context of the last entry, John Harley Warner, 'A Southern medical reform: the meaning of the antebellum argument for Southern medical education', *Bulletin of the History of Medicine*, 57 (1983), 364–81).

11. The difference in emphasis is especially evident in the testimony presented in the *Report from the Select Committee on Medical Education: With the Minutes of Evidence, and Appendix*, 4 vols (London: House of Commons, 1834).

12. 'Practice of physic', *Anderson's Quarterly Journal of Medical Science*, n.s. 1 (1824), 139–47, p. 140; 'Review of *Physiologie de l'Homme*, par N. P. Adelon', *Anderson's Quarterly Journal of Medical Science*, 2 (1825), 89–93, p. 90. And see 'The one faculty – instar omnium', *London Medical Gazette*, 13 (1833–4), 402–7, p. 406.

13. 'Medical reform in Germany', *London Medical Gazette*, 13 (1833–4), 723–7, p. 727.

14. Benjamin C. Brodie, *An Introductory Discourse, on the Studies Required for the Medical Profession. Addressed to the Students of the Medical School of St. George's Hospital, October 1, 1838* (London: T. Brettell, 1838), pp. 6–7; my emphasis. 'Although the medical men of the Continent receive a more elaborate scientific education than those of England, and have a more minute knowledge of morbid anatomy, that is, of disease, as an object of natural history,' another practitioner noted, 'yet there the superiority ends – while, as practitioners, they are as mere children, compared with the physicians and surgeons of England' ('Medical education in England', *London Medical Gazette*, 1 (1827–8), 10–11, p. 11).

15. The use of the decline argument by medical men engaged in scientific research is developed in Maulitz, *Morbid Appearances*. On the use of the argument to further provincial interests, see for example [William Sands Cox], *Remarks on the Importance of Extending the Means for the Cultivation of Medical Science in Birmingham, by One of the Lecturers of the School of Medicine* (Birmingham: J. C. Barlow, 1831), and '*An Address delivered to the Members of the Worcestershire Natural History Society, &c.*, By Charles Hastings, M.D.', *British Annals of Medicine*, 1 (1837), 656–7. Useful are Edward Mansfield Brockbank, *The Foundation of Provincial Medical Education in England and the Manchester School in Particular* (Manchester: Manchester University Press, 1936), and William H. McMenemy, *The Life and Times of Sir Charles Hastings*,

Founder of the British Medical Association (Edinburgh and London: E. & S. Livingstone Ltd., 1959).

16. J. G. Crosse to W. Worthington, Esq, FRSE, Norwich, 31 October 1846, in John Green Crosse, Letter Book, 1845–1846 (MS 472), Crosse Papers.

17. Irvine Loudon, *Medical Care and the General Practitioner 1750–1850* (Oxford: Clarendon Press, 1986); I. S. L. Loudon, 'The origin of the general practitioner', *Journal of the Royal College of General Practitioners*, 33, 246 (1963), 13–23. On professional structure and reform in English medicine, see S. W. F. Holloway, 'The Apothecaries' Act, 1815: a reinterpretation', *Medical History*, 10 (1966), 221–35; S.W.F. Holloway, 'Medical education in England, 1830–1858: a sociological analysis', *History*, 49 (1964), 299–324; Irvine Loudon, '"The Vile Race of Quacks With Which This Country is Infested"', in W. F. Bynum and Roy Porter (eds), *Medical Fringe and Medical Orthodoxy 1750–1850* (London: Croom Helm, 1987), pp. 106–28; Pauline M. H. Mazumdar, 'Anatomical physiology and the reform of medical education: London, 1825–1835', *Bulletin of the History of Medicine*, 57 (1983), 230–46; Charles Newman, *The Evolution of Medical Education in the Nineteenth Century* (London: Oxford University Press, 1957); M. Jeanne Peterson, *The Medical Profession in Mid-Victorian London* (Berkeley, Los Angeles and London: University of California Press, 1978); Matthew Ramsey, 'The politics of professional monopoly in nineteenth-century medicine: the French model and its rivals', in Gerald L. Geison (ed.), *Professions and the French State, 1700–1900* (Philadelphia: University of Pennsylvania Press, 1984), pp. 225–305; W. J. Reader, *Professional Men: The Rise of the Professional Classes in Nineteenth-Century England* (London: Weidenfeld & Nicolson, 1966); Edwina Sherrington, 'Thomas Wakley and reform, 1823–62' DPhil thesis, University of Oxford, 1973; Ivan Waddington, 'General practitioners and consultants in early nineteenth-century England: the sociology of an intra-professional conflict', in John Woodward and David Richards (eds), *Health Care and Popular Medicine in Nineteenth Century England* (London: Croom Helm, 1977), pp. 164–88; and Ivan Waddington, *The Medical Profession in the Industrial Revolution* (Dublin: Gill & Macmillan, 1984).

18. 'Comparative merits of French and English schools', *London Medical Gazette*, 19 (1836–7), 319–322, p. 319.

19. 'Anatomical report', *London Medical Gazette*, 2 (1828) 406–13, pp. 410, 411; and see 'Anatomy', *London Medical and Physical Journal*, 60 (1828), 373–83, and H. W. Rush, 'Clinical instruction in London and Paris', *Lancet*, 2 (1833–4), 321–2, p. 321.

20. 'Anatomy', *London Medical and Physical Journal*, 60 (1828), 373–83, pp. 378, 379.

21. 'Meeting of the medical profession at the Freemasons' Tavern', *London Medical and Surgical Journal*, n.s. 4 (1833–4), 376–7, p. 377. 'It is not the want of opportunity that renders our hospital physicians infinitely inferior to those of France as observers of disease, but the lack of *scientific enthusiasm* – a quality which, however, will never be found among them until the medical charities of this country are placed under other control than that which at present rules them,'

one reformer typically wrote in 1842. 'Our hospitals ought to be placed under the control of the Government, and the medical officers chosen by concours' ('Poverty of English medical literature', *Lancet*, 2 (1842–3), 197–9, pp. 197, 198).

22. William Baly to 'Dear Mother', London, 29 March [1834], William Baly Papers, Library, Royal College of Physicians. Baly was studying at St. Bartholomew's Hospital.

23. 'Defects of the London hospital system', *London Medical and Surgical Journal*, n.s. 7 (1835), 316–17, p. 316. This was hardly the perception of English students alone; compare the quoted remark and what an American medical student who had visited both Paris and London (and was about to cross the Channel again for Paris) wrote from London to his father in Boston: 'At Paris, I am to study under the influence of men whose aim is science – at London, gain' (James Jackson, Junior, to James Jackson, Senior, London, 12 September 1832, James Jackson Papers, Francis, A. Countway Library of Medicine, Boston, Massachusetts). And see 'Duties of public journalists', *Lancet*, 1 (1842–3), 134–7, and 'State of medicine in Italy', *London Medical and Physical Journal*, 61 (1829), 475–91, pp. 482–3.

24. 'The national system of medical education in France', *Medical Times*, 13 (1845–6), 37–9, p. 38.

25. 'Preface', *Lancet*, 1 (1838–9), 1–5, p. 2.

26. *Medical Times*, 14 (1846), 220.

27. *Medical Times*, 8 (1843), 90–3, p. 90.

28. See, for example, Report from the Court of Examiners to the Chairman of the Bill Committee, 11 June 1818, Act of Parliament Committee, Minutes, 1814–34 (Ms. 8211/1); Special Court of Assistants, 28 July 1821, and Court of Assistants, 1 August 1828, Court of Assistants, Minute Book, 1817–33 (Ms. 8200/11); and Report to the Court of Assistants, 21 July 1831, Court of Examiners, Minutes, vol. 4, 1828–33 (Ms. 8239/4), all in Society of Apothecaries Records, Guildhall Libary, London.

29. 'Causes of the depressed state of the medical profession in Great Britain', *Lancet*, 2 (1831–2), 88–92, pp. 88–9; *Medical Times*, 14 (1846), 220; 'Reform – College of Physicians', *London Medical Gazette*, 11 (1832–3), 485–9. 'Our medical corporations are composed of individuals who are placed there by interest, and not by scientific acquirements,' one critic commented ('Cholera in London, Dublin, and Paris', *London Medical and Surgical Journal*, n.s. 1 (1832), 440–3, p. 442).

30. 'Poverty of English medical literature', p. 197. And see 'Medical education in England', *London Medical Gazette*, 1 (1827–8), 10–11, p. 11, and 'Practice of physic', *Anderson's Quarterly Journal of Medical Sciences*, n.s. 1 (1824), 139–47, pp. 139–40.

31. 'Defects of the London hospital system', p. 316.

32. Dr. Brown, comments in 'Medical reform. Meeting of the North of England Medical Association', *Lancet*, 1 (1839–40), 737–9, p. 737.

33. Voyageur, 'Parisian news', letter to the editor, Paris, 1 May 1828, *London Medical Gazette*, 2 (1828), 695–7, p. 695.

34. Review of '*Durstellung und Ansichten zur Vergleichung der Medicin in Frankreich, England, und Deutchland, nach einer Reise in diesen Ländern im Jahre 1835.* Von Dr. Adolph Mühry', *British and Foreign Medical Review*, 3 (1837), 447–52, p. 449.

35. 'The National Association of General Practitioners', *Medical Times*, 13 (1845–6), 176–7, p. 176.

36. 'Dinner of medical practitioners. British Medical Association', *Lancet*, 1 (1836–7), 224–30, p. 226.

37. Edward Barlow to [Samuel Whitbread], Bath, 30 December 1813, in Samuel Whitbread Correspondence (4632), Bedfordshire County Record Office, County Hall, Bedford.

38. *Medical Times*, 8 (1843), 90–1, p. 90.

39. 'Medical reform – College of Physicians', *London Medical Gazette*, 10 (1832), 482–5, pp. 484, 485.

40. G. D. Dermott, 'The national system of medical education in France', *Medical Times*, 13 (1845–6), 37–9; 'Medicine *v.* government', *Medical Times*, 16 (1847), 497–8; 'Review of *An Essay on Clinical Instruction.* By E. Ch. A. Louis', *London Medical and Surgical Journal*, n.s. 6 (1835), 496–8. Critics forcefully pointed out that this was a highly idealized image of the French system; see, for example, 'The French schools', *Lancet*, 2 (1826–7), 699–701.

41. 'Depressed state of medical literature in England', *London Medical and Surgical Journal*, n.s. 6 (1835), 376–8, p. 377.

42. 'Corruption totters', *Lancet*, 2 (1830–1), 243–8, p. 245.

43. 'The incorporated general practitioners', *Lancet*, 2 (1844), 342–3, p. 342. This is his fuller comment: 'When we speak of the *medical profession of this country*, we wish it to be understood that we mean to embrace and define by that term . . . those practitioners who are engaged in discharging *all* the duties which belong to *physicians, surgeons*, and *apothecaries*. We refer, therefore, in using that term, to nineteen-twentieths of the profession; in a word, to the general practitioners in *medicine, surgery*, and *midwifery*. The *pure* physicians and *pure* surgeons, of all classes and degrees, are mere *offsets* from the great professional trunk, or parasites, which often exist to the great injury of the noble structure on which they have fastened.' And see 'Fundamental government of the profession', *Medical Times*, 5 (1841–2), 6–7; 'Medical reform', *Lancet*, 2 (1832–3), 255–6; and 'Preface', *Lancet*, 1 (1838–9), 1–5. And also see Ian Inkster, 'Marginal men: aspects of the social role of the medical community in Sheffield 1790–1850', in Woodward and Richards (eds), *Health Care and Popular Medicine*, pp. 128–63.

44. L. S. Jacyna, 'Images of John Hunter in the nineteenth century', *History of Science*, 21 (1983), 85–108.

45. J. G. Crosse, [Notes Taken on] Abernethy's Surgical Lectures, 20 January 1812 (MS 80), in Library, Royal Society of Medicine, London. And consider Astley Cooper's remarks outlining to pupils the knowledge necessary for surgeons four years later: 'Physiology is also necessary, as with out it you cannot be a Surgeon for it teaches the foundation of the profession, but to whom have we been indebted for this? To John Hunter, by some called hypothetical, but this is not the

case as he rather gave a mass of facts than drew conclusions from them and when he did draw from them, it was from what he had seen; Surgery before his time was good mechanical but after it good *scientific Surgery* [my emphasis] became founded in observation' (J. F. South, [Notes Taken on] Lectures on the Principles and Practice of Surgery delivered by Astley Paston Cooper Esq F.R.S. & Benjamin Travers Esq FRS in the Anatomical Theatre at St Thomas's Hospital between the years 1816 & 1818, vol. 1, A. P. Cooper, Introductory Lecture, 5 October 1816 (275.b.15), in Library, Royal College of Surgeons). Benjamin Brodie was typical of later élite surgeons in casting 'the science connected with our profession' in the tradition of Hunter; see B. C. Brodie to J. H. James, London, 18 September 1821, James Papers (64/8/8/9).

46. 'Narrative of a journey to London, in 1814, . . . *By* Philibert Joseph Roux', *Monthly Medico-Chirurgical Review and Chemico-Philosophical Magazine*, n.s. 1 (1824), 156–9, 202–8, p. 202.

47. 'Medical reform', *Lancet*, 1 (1837–8), 489–92, p. 491.

48. The tension between an accountability to science and to the maintenance of gentlemanly values in defining professional identity and conferring status was, of course, exceptionally durable, and though altered it persisted in many ways unresolved at least through the first decades of the twentieth century.

49. The development of this point in the historiography of American medicine is reviewed in John Harley Warner, 'Science in medicine', in Sally Gregory Kohlstedt and Margaret W. Rossiter (eds), *Historical Writing on American Science: Perspectives and Prospects* (Baltimore and London: Johns Hopkins University Press, 1986), pp. 37–58. On science in England, see Morris Berman, *Social Change and Scientific Organization: The Royal Institution, 1799–1844* (London: Heinemann, 1978); D. S. L. Cardwell, *The Organisation of Science in England* (London: Heinemann, 1957); T. W. Heyck, *The Transformation of Intellectual Life in Victorian England* (London: Croom Helm, 1982), pp. 13–22, 50–154; and the essays in Ian Inkster and Jack Morrell (eds), *Metropolis and Province: Science in British Culture 1780–1850* (Philadelphia: University of Pennsylvania Press, 1983). On the place and persistent ambiguities of the language of science in English medicine, see Stella V. F. Butler, 'Science and medicine in the nineteenth century: changing conceptions of clinical practice', paper presented 19 April 1985 at conference on Science in Medicine, Manchester; Christopher Lawrence 'Incommunicable knowledge: science and the clinical art 1850–1914', *Journal of Contemporary History*, 20 (1985), 503–20; Irvine Loudon, 'The concept of the family doctor', *Bulletin of the History of Medicine*, 58 (1984), 347–62; Peterson, *Medical Profession in Mid-Victorian London*; and S. E. D. Shortt, 'Physicians, science, and status: issues in the professionalization of Anglo-American medicine in the nineteenth century', *Medical History*, 27 (1983), 51–68.

50. Granville not only actively used the declinist theme in urging medical reform, but also was an active player in Babbage's decline-of-science controversy; see his *Science without a Head; or, the Royal Society Dissected* (London: T. Ridgway, 1830). And see 'British Medical

Association', *Lancet*, 2 (1840–1), 83–97, and 'Medical reform', *Lancet*, 2 (1832–3), 255–6.

51. The portrayal of science by those who championed the general practitioners in the decline-of-science rhetoric might also be profitably compared with the portrayal of science in the languages of other medical cultures within English society, such as those of élite physicians or surgeons and of adherents to the botanical medical sect, Coffinism.

52. The place of French medicine in American medical practitioners' programmes for professional reform is discussed in John Harley Warner, 'The selective transport of medical knowledge: antebellum American physicians and Parisian medical therapeutics', *Bulletin of the History of Medicine*, 59 (1985), 213–31, and in John Harley Warner, *The Therapeutic Perspective: Medical Practice, Knowledge, and Identity in America, 1820–1885* (Cambridge, Mass., and London: Harvard University Press, 1986), pp. 37–57, 185–206. On the rooting of American professional identity in practice, see John Harley Warner, 'Medical sectarianism, therapeutic conflict, and the shaping of orthodox professional identity in antebellum American medicine', in Bynum and Porter (eds), *Medical Fringe and Medical Orthodoxy*, pp. 234–60. A fuller comparative study of the use American and English reformers made of the French medical model is in process.

53. The idea of science that the Americans and the English presented in this reformist rhetoric made no necessary or consistent reference to any particular body of natural knowledge. Obviously, individual examples of the vitality of French medical science often pointed to a particular body of knowledge (especially pathological anatomy), as did their Anglo-American foils. Yet all such specific references could just as easily fall away when reformers spoke about something broader that was science. This much the Americans and the English shared.

54. The present study urges a more sensitive re-reading of the language of science that became so prominent in medicine during the final decades of the nineteenth century. Historians have rightly given considerable attention to the use of the rhetoric of science as a cultural tool in late-nineteenth and early-twentieth-century medical professionalization. Yet they have tended to regard this as something new. On the contrary, a loudly proclaimed allegiance to science was neither new nor simply newly prominent. What needs to be closely scrutinized is how the idea of science that was represented in medical language changed and, similarly, how the intellectual and social locus of those within the profession who deployed science in their reformist rhetoric changed. Such an analysis could do historiographic service by going beyond the simple proposition that medicine became more scientific during the nineteenth century to show how the meaning of science in medicine changed.

7

Why were most medical heretics at their most confident around the 1840s? (The other side of mid-Victorian medicine)

Logie Barrow

Unlike the others in this volume, this chapter will examine opposition to the consolidating 'orthodox' medical profession and to those doctrines and practices associated with it. At the legal level, the consolidation climaxed with the 1858 Medical Act. The doctrines and practices centred on massive interventions directed, accurately or not, at particular parts or areas of the body. Those readers for whom the first sentence of this chapter remains abstract are referred to much of the rest of this book as well as to later on in this chapter. To ignore the opponents of orthodoxy is not merely to commit 'enormous condescension' towards them but also, more important, to suppress the very relationship of opposition, and thus to smother the light it can throw on what was being opposed. Even those historians who – from beyond the pale of this volume, surely – still insist on interrogating the past for pioneers of a more or less triumphally viewed modernity need to keep alive some curiosity as to what their heroes (and, exceptionally, heroines) were up against.

As is now well known, the generation or so from the 1830s onwards saw in Britain a growth of movements – some observers said sects – of medical opposition. A list might include hydropathy, homoeopathy, mesmerism, phreno-mesmerism, spiritual healing, medical botany, and its derivative (more or less) 'eclecticism'. But this list is not necessarily exhaustive – not least because these tendencies combined fresh elements with older ones. The older ones came from the, to us, historiographically hazy area which we label 'folk medicine', and their practitioners did not form any movement. In addition, those who offered one or other securely delimitable type of medical assistance within the field of medicine often – as Roger Cooter[1] has pointed out in relation to bonesetting – continued or in effect negotiated a more or less amicable coexistence with the medically qualified orthodox.

No relationship, whether of opposition or of coexistence, can be grasped in terms of one side alone. There is thus much value in the contrast drawn by Porter and others between the relatively undifferentiated and easy-going eighteenth century and the more polarized generations after about 1790. There may also be some heuristic value in turning the issue round and enquiring to what extent orthodoxy was the side which gave the most impulse towards sectarianization. Were *this* pattern to be substantiated, it might be thought to make Britain the inverse of the USA, where orthodoxy continued to be much weaker throughout the nineteenth century and where, at least according to John Harley Warner,[2] orthodox doctors were therefore reduced to behaving in ways as sect-like as their opponents. But this contrast is too static – not least here, because the intellectual balance within the British Isles was to shift decisively to orthodoxy's advantage between, say, the 1840s and around 1900.

Not that oppositional movements may strike us as enjoying intellectual stability either. Within virtually every one of the movements listed two paragraphs above, successive or even contemporaneous practitioners claimed to be offering fundamental innovations (or revivals of buried truth). That many of these claimed to harmonize with one another only added to the general confusion. Whatever the din, though, most of these movements had some features in common.[3] For one thing, whatever their differences, they were holistic, in two senses. First, each tended to reduce all complaints to its particular fundament (as summarily as possible: hydropathy to disturbances of heat in the body; homoeopathy and medical botany to disturbances of the normal balance of bodily fluids; mesmerism to disharmonies with the cosmic fluid; phreno-mesmerism to such disharmonies as were supposedly accessible via stimulation or relaxation of particular parts of the cranium; eclecticism to some, most often mainly medico-botanic, mixture of these, sometimes as diagnosed and cured by 'spiritual healing', i.e. with the aid of dematerialized spirits). Second, each tended thereby to treat the body as an interactive whole which was also psychosomatic: the mind (however defined) was part of such interaction.

Third, many of them were involved in what I have elsewhere dubbed the problematic of imponderables; within this, briefly, the less traceable a substance, the more powerful it might be argued to be. A 'substance' might be a medicine (particularly if refined to a homoeopathic subtlety) or, say, the 'mesmeric fluid' or a 'spiritual body' or indeed anything imaginable as operating near borders where superfine materiality might shade into alleged immaterial entities. As I have argued in the same place, this problematic is as old as Newton – or rather, as the various readings or misreadings of him during the eighteenth century. But, by the nineteenth, it often came clothed in a jargon of vital fluids which was particularly handy for bringing these heresies into harmony.[4] 'Disease', declared an 1857 editorial in the *Homoeopathic Record*, 'is not some distinct entity capable of being hunted after through muscle, blood, nerve and tissue and, when met with, poisoned *right out* with pill and bolus.' Rather, 'every form of disease' originated as a disturbance to 'the balance between the physical and the spiritual man'. Under such disturbance,

> the brain will either secrete too large or too small a quantity of the nervo-vital fluid, or there will be a mal distribution [sic] of that which is normally generated. From the nature of the case, the recuperative agent will be found among the '*imponderabilia*' in some form or other. The remedy must be infinitesimal in its action . . . in order that vital electricity, the connecting link between the spirit-form and the body-man, may act upon it. Since that which is acted upon are structures and forms of an evanescent character, the remedies . . . must of necessity be of the same class of agencies.

The 'artificial' among the latter included, for this editorial, not merely homoeopathic medicines, but also 'the mesmeric pass', and the 'infusion of the galvanic fluid, or the decomposition of the vital electricity by the same agency', by means of 'the electric shock'. All these means owed their effectiveness to 'their imponderable nature'.[5]

But, fourth, their imponderably based holism went with something more important. Supporters of oppositional types of medication often claimed something more than curativeness superior to that of the orthodox. Rather, they attributed this superiority to what they saw as a fundamentally better relationship with patients. Orthodox approaches were seen as doing violence to patients, oppositional ones as working with them. This claim was particularly clear from homoeopaths, but could also be heard, dubiously or not, from medical botanists, eclectics, and mesmerists. Oppositionals often seem to have believed that they listened to patients more than their orthodox rivals did. Again, whether or not such claims were always accurate, they were consistent with a holistic approach. Of course, when listening, the unorthodox had a supposedly superior interpretative apparatus. And in other ways, too, the communication could be far from equal. Aside from any differences of class and gender, a spiritual healer would claim some kind of occult knowledge, and mesmerists would allegedly be in a different state of consciousness from their 'subjects' during the most distinctive stage of the treatment.

Fifth, and no less important, bonesetting, hydropathy, mesmerism, spiritual healing, and perhaps even eclecticism involved the practitioner manipulating, using hands and perhaps arms – and, with mesmerism notoriously, eyes. Such manipulations varied in scope, direction, speed, or strength from heresy to heresy or even (what is presumably uncheckable) from heretic to heretic. The point is that – apart, usually, from bonesetting – they sometimes involved (and, in mesmerism, necessitated) a belief that such use worked with or via some fluid within and/or outside the physical body.

Indeed, sixth, a few heterodox approaches – not all, by any means – involved elements of some variety of what today might be called transference between sufferer and healer,[6] during which healers supposedly distanced the problem from the sufferer, sometimes by in some sense sharing it temporarily themselves. This was most often so with 'spiritual healing'. Obviously, the last three aspects went well with the allegations that orthodox practitioners were indifferent or cold.

Altogether, the din of novelty or apparent novelty involved much repetition and (as we have seen with the *Homoeopathic Record*) overlap. These related to another very common denominator which I have called the epistemological. This word is here taken from – or rather out of – strictly philosophical discourse in order to supply a grammatically flexible link between particular social groupings on the one hand and their often clashing views as to the accessibility of particular bodies of knowledge (or alleged knowledge) on the other. In this sense, everyone is an epistemologist just as everyone usually speaks prose: epistemological assumptions – about such things as potential or actual ability, incapability, comprehensibility, availability, and, say, agendability – form a little-discussed foundation to many aspects of life, prosaic or otherwise. The period and field which form the subject of this chapter were epistemologically among the liveliest or most polarized in British history at least. This was partly because most of our oppositionals in all the fields listed in our second paragraph (with the exceptions we are about to make among some homoeopaths and mesmerists) held vocally to a democratic epistemology. Their knowledge (as they saw it) was open to the open-minded, irrespective of class or education. For them, the falsity of official medicine and its (often, as we are about to see, no less vocal), epistemological élitism reinforced each other.

True, the phrase 'most . . . oppositionals' is there to allow of many exceptions. One type would be those of the regularly qualified homoeopaths who wished to establish the respectability of their approach, not merely by accumulating posh patients and supporters, but also by doing everything possible to separate themselves from those homoeopaths unable (or, in some cases, unwilling)[7] to acquire regular qualifications: the F.H.H. Quins, we might say, as against the Spencer T. Halls (though how typical either of these extreme cases is of those calling themselves homoeopaths remains unclear even from the latest full-scale study of the subject).[8] Another type would be those believers in mesmerism who, precisely because they believed it could be practised by almost anyone, preferred to keep such practice in the 'right' hands – whether those of gentlemen exclusively, or ladies too, and/or clergy of one's own or sympathetic denominations – for fear that it might be misused for socially or sexually undesirable ends.[9] Dr John Elliotson is a good instance here. From 1838 he was very much mesmerism's most august martyr for having – rather than discontinue his mesmeric activities – sacrificed his professorship of the theory and practice of medicine at London's University College Hospital (an institution in whose founding he had been prominent).

Conversely, when we talk of the epistemology of most oppositionals being democratic, we must also note that, all too often, it boiled down (once the rhetoric had evaporated) to a democracy based on shared allegiance, real or assumed, to certain presuppositions. To this extent, such democracy was sectarian. Minimally, these presuppositions were about epistemology and imponderables, if not, more narrowly, about one or other version of, say, medical botany – as between the followers of Dr Coffin or of the eclectic, John Skelton. Organizations were of variable tightness. With botanics and eclectics at least, the main unit was always the local face-to-face gathering of part-timers, overwhelmingly working and lower-middle class. Coffinites – or Coffin at least – would probably have wanted some grander discipline. They were laughed at by eclectics for this, and seem not to have achieved much durable organization. Skelton's followers, on their side, made only spasmodic efforts. Apparently these were not very fruitful as compared with the models being emulated (variously: union, temperance, friendly society, Methodist, or the Yorkshire Union of Mechanics' Institutes). None the less, the mid-Victorian decades did see organizations such as the National Medical Reform League, which was conceived and launched during 1853–4 with twenty-five local secretaries, who hailed disproportionately from Northern England, or, later, the British Medical Reform Association. By the 1860s there was also the 'School of Domestic Medicine' being run by Skelton's son in Bloomsbury, London, and, from 1869, an 'Eclectic School of Medicine' in Leeds, which enrolled its first intake of 'nearly forty'.[10] These latter were all described as 'gentlemen': almost certainly, the drive for organization – which could easily become one for respectability – restricted the visibility of women below their continued level of involvement in at least herbal medicine.

As for the homoeopaths, the 1850s and 1860s were their period of maximum optimism and of no less panic and sectarianism among their orthodox opponents. One aspect of this flowed precisely from the influence and financial pull of the more up-market homoeopaths and was manifested in their founding of hospitals – more often on a sound financial footing than any medico-botanic foundation – as also of journals and dispensaries. Indeed, in one or two centres such dispensaries may have enjoyed significant multi-class support (assuming we can trust the claim by a homoeopathic periodical that 500 persons had attended the 1856 annual meeting, chaired by the heterodox baronet Sir Charles Isham, of the Northampton

Homoeopathic Dispensary).[11] By contrast, botany was well adapted to pursuit by poor people. Anyone with legs to take them to the local countryside or with the friendship of like-minded collectors of local and other herbs was potentially a dispenser, with or without dispensary or any kind of official dispensation.

Yet, even had the homoeopaths' organizational achievement been as fitful and patchy as that of, say, botanists and eclectics, it would still have underlined a major contrast with the eighteenth century: an orthodoxy and some heterodoxies were defining themselves and each other, not only doctrinally but also organizationally. Admittedly, some other heterodoxies seem to have remained more loosely structured, when not virtually unorganized. But part of the argument of this chapter is that epistemological dimensions can often be found haunting ones that are historiographically more familiar. I say 'often' because few hauntings are continuously discernible. To continue, here, with organization: many partisans, of unorganized and semiorganized heterodoxies alike, tended to draw strength from fresh variations on the biblical epistemology that knowledge came more directly to the intellectually humble than to the mightily qualified.

These assumptions were no doubt far older than the mid-seventeenth-century interregnum, when they had surfaced with unmistakable splashings. On the other hand, the Porters have recently compared the 'medical ideas and information' of the 'long 18th century' to 'one continuous ocean, partially divided up here and there into seas, bays and straits'. The contrast with what emerged during the nineteenth century is thus clearer than ever. However, in explaining this contrast, the same authors plausibly gesture towards the peculiar weakness of England's state as against civil society during the one hundred and eighty or so years from the mid-seventeenth century. During these, nationally intrusive structures of state-backed corporate control were impossible. The contrast is also geographical: with those Continental countries (nearly all) whose states were more or less absolutist and where, the implication is, such structures did emerge. Now, admittedly, the Porters do mention other factors as important, such as the sheer prosperity and sophistication of the medical market (among consumers as much as providers) in Britain as compared, apparently, with those on the Continent. But this itself comes to seem causatively no more than an aspect of the flourishing of an un-statified civil society.[12]

Thus any extra-terrestrial reader knowledgeable on medical but ignorant on political history might imagine that the 'long 18th century' formed merely a long interregnum between the failed absolutism of Charles I or Cromwell and the triumphant absolutism of Victoria and her consort, Edwin of Saxe-Coburg-Chadwick. And it so happens that many of the nineteenth century's losers – from opponents of anything from workhouse 'Bastilles' to vaccination – would have applauded our extra-terrestrial in this (the anti-vaccinationists till at least the end of the century when they ceased being automatic losers). For them, the behaviour of the state and/or of the medical profession-as-by-law-enthroned was essentially absolutist and thereby 'un-English'. For them, the nature of the 'revolution in government' to which they were being subjected was no matter for mid-twentieth-century historians alone.

And yet, particularly if one can at least argue that Chartists helped undermine their movement by clinging to an obsolete theory of the state,[13] one can also be allowed to see analogous if equally understandable mistakes being made by many medical oppositionists too. Even if we were to see the rise of Whitehall as merely a mutation in an older absolutism of Westminster,[14] orthodox medicine was so variably absolute that 'the number of herbalists listed in Manchester Directories' (reliably or not) could grow 'from two in 1852 to 171 in 1891, most of them in working-class areas.'[15]

Altogether, whether or not the Porters are fully correct about the long eighteenth century, the changes from this to the mid-nineteenth century had dimensions more numerous than a mere relation between state and society. Though this relation may have considerable explanatory mileage, its effects were not organizational alone. The relation itself also had an epistemological dimension. Here we can hardly be surprised that so many would-be democratic practitioners and self-medictors, whose forebears the long eighteenth century had accustomed to splashing around in the Porters' global ocean of medical knowledge (whether as, say, bewigged seahorses or humble sardines), refused to submit tamely to being herded by the 1858 Medical Act and others into backwaters, there to be intellectually stranded if not legally gutted.

The epistemological dimension extended far beyond the medical field, however. Tensions over the accessibility and, therewith, definition of knowledge were diffuse enough to surface through the nineteenth and into the early twentieth century at least, in many a field from, say, Mechanics' Institutes to university extension to elementary schooling[16] to avowed class struggle (as in the 1909 Ruskin College strike and the ensuing Labour Colleges movement). In the long run, and very much with hindsight, we can assume that, from around the 1870s or 1880s, a larger proportion of the population than before was prepared to accord established definitions of medical knowledge the benefit of any doubt. The significance of orthodox medicine around the 1840s, though, is that the process of its becoming established preceded most of the main curative breakthroughs of these two centuries, in other words, came at a time when orthodox medicine enjoyed at best uncertain intellectual prestige. (That the latter was merely the other side of the coin to low social prestige was obvious to orthodoxy's main journalistic strategists, as we shall see.) Indeed, given that orthodoxy was still in the throes of being born, we may be forgiven for mixing our metaphors and saying that it was born out on a limb: by definition a convoluted process. We can begin to understand, therefore, why medicine was such an embattled area of epistemological relations during much of the nineteenth century.

We can also understand better why a do-it-yourself attitude to medication remained strong among very many people, perhaps particularly among the poor. But similar attitudes also flourished outside the area of medication. In some of these areas, spare-time practitioners could at least hope – and, even around mid-century, still not always illusorily – to be taken seriously by even the 'greatest' or most established of professionals or gentlemen-virtuosi. We have only to think of the naturalist A. R. Wallace. And for every Wallace there was also a second category: self-taught plebeian enthusiasts such as Robert Dick, the walking baker-geologist of Thurso, or Thomas Edwards, the shoemaker-naturalist who became an Associate of the Linnaean Society. These two were at least known outside their localities. More numerous, however, were members of a third category who might plausibly aspire (though almost always vainly) to become like the Dicks in some field or other. At the local level, such people might enjoy some Dick-like reputation.[17]

Plebeians and established scientists might hold very various views on other matters of importance to them, such as politics or religion. The point, however – the main point of the remaining pages – is merely that the unevenness and sometimes openness of the epistemological situation in many areas away from medicine was often seen, however implicitly, as contrasting with that which was developing – and being brought about – within or near the medical field.

And this highlights a quality which we can associate with the generations around roughly 1800. Even if, as late as the first half of the nineteenth century, there was still no 'single orthodoxy', let alone 'single "fringe"',[18] we are told that the eighteenth century had seen very little firm division between any orthodoxy and any fringe – possibly to the extent that, as Michael Neve has recently ironized, the historiography of eighteenth-century 'quackery' is 'in danger of losing its object' with 'the ultimate quack' becoming 'the consumer patient'.[19] As against such a past, the situation was clarifying – the Apothecaries' Act of 1815 is now generally seen as marking the start of a process in which the medical profession was legally allowed to define itself nationally, i.e. at far more than a mere few miles' radius from Charing Cross. But this view would have probably felt glib to the mass of medical practitioners who felt increasingly hard-pressed between the power of the old élitist Royal Colleges on the one hand and, on the other, the seemingly growing popularity and even influence of quacks of all classes. Thus the 1840s and 1850s saw mounting agitation among medical practitioners to allow them to control not only admission to their ranks but also to ban any practice felt to discredit them as, they hoped, a coming profession. Thus, the pressure increased to define heresies and to hunt out, brand, and ostracize heretics. Into and through the 1850s, there were even calls to enshrine an orthodox pharmacopoeia in law and thus make any use of drugs or treatments excluded from it or denounced in it into a punishable offence. This pressure enjoyed no direct success. But, in general, one crucial criterion for rejecting many a practice or medication as heretical was that it seemed easy for the uninitiated to learn or administer – or, worse, that its adherents even proclaimed this. All these pressures were irrespective of the medical behaviour of some or perhaps many individual practitioners in the localities, let alone irrespective of whether any of them held, as individuals, a democratic view of knowledge. Moreover, during the same generations, orthodox practitioners were also intervening once more, often backed by public authorities, notably via sanitary measures, public health, and, as we shall see, vaccination. As is notorious, the terms of this backing – not to mention the relations between the various medical bodies – were fraught with controversy: this was what animated medical reformers, not least Thomas Wakley and the *Lancet*. But Wakley was as aware as anyone that his whole project (which was to come to, for him, so stunted a fruition in the 1858 Medical Act) depended not only on defining orthodoxy as based on the natural sciences but also, no less, on utterly excluding the unqualified (let alone patients) from this basis. These two projects were one, even to the exclusion of otherwise potential allies such as the wealthier and more scientistic of the druggists.[20]

Wakley thus demands greater vigilance than he normally receives. He is often seen as a democrat and meritocrat. True, on a broadly political canvas, most issues found him more attuned to popular feeling than almost any MP, not least because he shared a widespread popular contempt for aristocracy and ascriptive tradition. Even here, though, he was not nearly as warm towards Chartism as his fellow medical-reforming MP Thomas Duncombe. And here there may also be relevance in Duncombe's much greater sympathy for medical heresies – or, at the very least, for homoeopathy and medical botany. For, likewise on the medical canvas, Wakley was certainly a democrat for those he recognized as the rank-and-file of the profession he was seeking to redesign – and a meritocrat thereby. But, when meritocrats are democrats, they are so on one absolute precondition: that they define merit. Thus the democratic qualities of Wakley's whole project for a powerfully functionalized medical profession were hedged about with conceptual and epistemological sneerings, fumigations, and excommunications: meritocracy too may have its sectarian aspects.

'In 19th-century England and America', 'gut distrust' among patients and lay people towards the more orthodox of medicators can be said, as by Porter,[21] to have 'belched forth'. In many places, this symptom continued for at least the rest of the century; whether the complaint itself had altered is another matter. Sweepingly, we can say that, in the early nineteenth century, much of the medical profession was confronted with a number of problems – *wholly* new, such as cholera, about which it was generally agreed to have covered itself in confusion in 1832 and arguably also during the long-anticipated but still more devastating outbreak of 1848–9; or *partly* new, such as the problems associated with the spread or intensification of what we would call industrialization and urbanization.

At the same time, many a method in more routine situations was so radical in its dosages as to be likely to heighten routine into something more precarious. Certainly, one should not distort the decline of this so-called 'heroic' medicine – a decline whose speed varied – into a simple story of patients' disgust. But violent dosages – even when expected or even welcomed – were likely to be high-profile. So, presumably, once patients and those nearest to them or surviving them *had* grown to distrust such methods, this distrust might become anger when peppered with memories, let alone with further experiences, however indirect, of apparent ineptitude of a 'heroic' type.

Not only in their methods (or in memories of them) is the adjective 'high-profile' appropriate to the position of orthodox doctors: rather, it needs applying in area after area. We might, for example, cite the struggles before and particularly after the 1832 Anatomy Act,[22] or the long agitation culminating in the 1858 Act. But the point is that, in this agitation, doctors were – because of all these aspects – epistemologically out on a limb and striving for a position in which their legal reach was widely seen as exceeding their curative grasp.

All this helps us to understand why no less astute a strategist than Wakley viewed, not with joy but with panic, the heightening of a further exclusive role for his designated profession, the – admittedly at first not very effective – legislation, in 1853, for compulsory vaccination. His arguments, coming from one with a sometimes superb instinct for the strategic situation, surely illuminate this. 'In the public mind extensively, and to a more limited extent in the profession itself,' he warned,

> doubts are known to exist on the efficacy . . . of vaccination. The failures of the operation have been too numerous and discouraging. . . . Many a parent, of high and low degree, dates constitutional disease in her offspring to vaccination with 'bad matter'. Who shall say that this etiological [sic] conclusion is always false? . . . The poor are told that they must carry their children to be vaccinated by medical men who are strangers to them. They apprehend

– and the apprehension is not altogether unfounded or unshared by the educated classes – that the vaccine matter employed may carry with it the seeds of other diseases not less loathsome than the one it is intended to prevent. . . . So widely extended is the dread that along with the prophylactic remedy, something else may be innoculated, diseases may be implanted, that few medical practitioners would care to vaccinate their own children from a source of the purity of which they were not well assured.[23]

Wakley's basic line here – and one still shared by many who, otherwise, disagreed with him fundamentally, such as many an established homoeopath – was that vaccination was very good when properly done ('the greatest boon,' said he, 'that science ever gave mankind')[24] but that compulsion would be catastrophic. Wakley warned that an increase in compulsion would, very likely, 'bring vaccination into unmerited and irrecoverable disgrace' and, even worse, prove 'suicidal' for 'the [medical] profession'.[25]

The reasons which he gave for his pessimism group themselves under two headings. First, compulsion would wreck what he liked to see as a relationship of trust between doctor and poor patient. (Naturally, he did not stop here to wonder how far any such trust might depend on a doctor's being more flexible on both payment and medical doctrine than the *Lancet* would normally have tolerated.) This was because, even more centrally, the machinery for enforcement was already in the hands of Poor Law Guardians. Wealthier parents would usually pay for the operation to be done by their regular doctor, whose dexterity, and, more important, whose judgement as to the purity of the vaccine-lymph, they themselves might trust. Poorer parents would often receive no such reassurance: mass vaccination was by whomever the Guardians had appointed as public vaccinator. Wakley had led many a fight of doctors against Guardians, and he now reminded his readers that the latter were also 'too often looked upon with the greatest distrust by the poor'.[26]

Second, much debatable lymph was indeed in circulation; Wakley, for one, was 'certain' that it had 'been extensively used'. True, he could try to blame some of his customary scapegoats, and more plausibly than on many occasions: the stuff had 'in many instances . . . been put into circulation by benevolent clergymen and ladies, and even crones and midwives, who took it upon themselves to vaccinate the poor' – a typically ageist, anti-clerical, anti-feminist, anti-snob and (with the word 'even') anti-plebeian selection of his pet hates. But his overall prediction was already plausible and, during subsequent decades, was to appear far more so – often all too correctly. Compulsion would modify not only the grounds for popular distrust of orthodox medicators but also, among all classes, receptivity to the image of orthodoxy purveyed by medical dissenters such as homoeopaths and medical botanists.

The comprehensiveness of Wakley's sneers brings us to a threat which he had been loudly and lengthily denouncing since 1837, that of mesmerism. Mesmerism has been argued, as by Terry Parssinen, to have fallen foul of Wakley and others 'because it seemed to place one person so totally in the power of another' and because of its openness to mystical interpretations.[27] Certainly, overtones of hysteria about social and sexual subversion were present in Wakley's and similar polemics. But mesmerism did not automatically encourage mysticism. Thus, though Elliotson himself was to end as a Christian believer in spiritualism (1868), the Phrenological Association of London, which he dominated, celebrated his 1842 birthday with a materialist eulogy to phreno-mesmerism from his fellow-mesmerist W. C. Engledue; and Elliotson later contributed a preface to the printed version where Engledue attacked idealism in science as 'a malignant disease, which [could] only be cured by extermination'.[28] Engledue saw clairvoyance too as grist to his materialist mill.[29] In other words, imponderables frightened Wakley and others, not always because of any built-in bias towards mysticism but rather, sometimes at least, because of a deeper instability which could encourage almost any extreme philosophical position or lurchings between such.

Further, the imponderable and the epistemological aspects are often hard to disentangle, and the latter often lay at the root of the social fears. This was because the effects of mesmerism were often, perhaps potentially always, untraceable – unlike those of material anaesthetics. Thus, when opponents of mesmerism trumpeted instances of its sexual misuse, defenders were missing the point when they answered simply with a 'you too', to the effect that instances existed of no less scandalous misuse of physical anaesthetics. Rather – mesmeric fluid or no

– mesmerism's immateriality (or ultra-fine materiality, depending on one's metaphysical crotchet) helped make it peculiarly elusive in the face of non-mesmeric attempts to monitor, not its social or sexual subversiveness alone, but its mere effectiveness. The elusiveness was part of the underlying reason for mesmerism's being denounced – in Parssinen's nice quotation from the 1844 *London Medical Gazette* – for 'enabl[ing] the veriest dunderhead to go hand-in-hand, as a "philosophical inquirer" (forsooth!) with men of the highest scientific repute!',[30] or even more menacingly, as by Wakley, for allowing 'the ignorant and foolish of the laity [to] become the judges of what ought to be a learned and scientific profession'.[31] The latter vision amounted to a return with a vengeance of a degree of patient power much wider even than that which some historians identify with the eighteenth century. Thus, whether or not any visions of wholesale mesmeric undermining of society were ever set down in full – as opposed to being hinted at, more or less hysterically – mesmerism's main directly subversive potential was seen, surely with considerable justification, as what I have called epistemological (which, after all, is no more than what Robert Darnton has noted for it in France during the pre-Revolutionary years).[32]

Thus, for all these reasons, most ideologists of mesmerism (though, as noted with Engledue, not all) and those of a would-be scientific medicine, while not going out of their way to attack each other, were often correct in perceiving themselves as already on a collision course. This was why compromisers – even those as august as Sir John Forbes – tended to be squeezed out. Forbes had pleaded in the *Lancet* as late as 1844 that 'mesmerism [and similarly clairvoyance] may be true, though its professors are false' and, more broadly, in his *British and Foreign Medical Review*, in favour of what he dubbed the 'pseudo-sciences', that 'though they have no truth in them they generally have some truth *under* them'. In 1847, his tolerance drove his *Review* out of existence.[33] This often confrontational situation is surely behind the swift ripplings of excitement from late 1846 over ether and, soon, chloroform in anaesthetics. These, or at least the ripplings, allowed an end to the situation in which orthodoxy could be represented as callous about pain, where some of those it scorned as 'quacks' claimed to offer relief. Indeed it allowed the tables to be turned on 'quackery', in that those religious fundamentalists who defended pain as God-given were soon switching their main fire from mesmerists to physical anaesthetics, thus enhancing orthodoxy's scientific image all the more. Representation was here even more important than actuality: some orthodox continued to see pain as therapeutic, particularly for women, and there remained occasional cases where doctors laid themselves open to charges of extreme callousness, as with the more-than-twelve-hour flagellation of the feet of Augustus Stafford MP in 1857.[34]

We can glimpse how far Wakley, for one, was prepared to emphasize representation as compared with actuality from possibly the longest editorial which even he ever penned against mesmerism. Symbolically for my argument, it chanced to be printed less than four months before the famous Massachusetts demonstration which launched ether and soon chloroform on their world careers,[35] and was occasioned by Elliotson's being invited (even though merely by the customary principle of rotation) to give the Harveian Oration of the Royal College of Physicians.

Why did Wakley see mesmerism as 'this worst leprosy' and thus denounce the whole occasion as 'expos[ing] the members of the profession to the contagion of one tainted by' it? Centrally because Harvey, for him, represented the root of orthodoxy's claim to scientificity. Thus Elliotson, the great pariah, was about to defile the grand totem. Many aspects of this editorial have been quoted elsewhere,[36] not least the accusations against mesmerism of blasphemy and formlessness. But Wakley reached his rhetorical climax – we might say, anachronistically, his *Pseuds' Corner* – with a lachrymose description of his visit, allegedly a few days previously, to 'the tomb of the immortal discoverer of the circulation of the blood'. Here, 'we bent with reverence over the mortal remains of the most noble nature that has ever belonged to the profession of medicine. In the rustic church . . . ' etc. This nobility was not merely because, as Wakley capitalized, 'BACON DESCRIBED THE METHOD, HARVEY EXECUTED THE FIRST GREAT PROBLEM'. Rather, 'the noble characteristic of Harvey lay in his love of his profession'. And why did the two go together? Medicine, Wakley complained, remained no more than a 'noble, godlike and beneficent art'; now, though,

> the profession must become scientific; it must cease to be mere empiricism. . . . We must follow the track of the

> other and more certain sciences, in their march from what the great French philosopher, M. Comte, calls the superstitious ages of knowledge to the ages of *certain* and *fixed* science. We must imitate, not only *Tycho Brahe* and *Galileo* the great discoverers of *facts*, but we must follow *Kepler* and *Newton*, the discoverers of *laws* and *principles*. We must observe facts in medicine, subject the objects of medicine to our glasses, to deduce laws, and to detect principles of action. The mere observer, the 'mere practical man', must yield to the scientific practitioner.[37]

In the loudness, let alone in the manner in which he summoned the dominant philosophies of science to his side, Wakley was adding to the plausibility with which the heterodox viewed orthodoxy as inherently intolerant and no less inherently callous: might not patients – particularly poor and female ones – be among those entities ('objects of medicine') to be 'subject to our glasses'? It was crystal clear here who was supposed to be focusing judgement on whom. Subsequent years and decades were to furnish examples of both intolerance and callousness.

But, for us, the interest of Wakley – not least, as here, at his most purple – is the enormity of his demands in relation to the actual achievement of any such scientific medicine in most fields by June 1846. If orthodoxy was not the deadly confidence-trick its foes often alleged it to be, it was all too often open to being represented as requiring a very long-term *lending* of confidence – perhaps with repayment dates falling some indefinite time after the lender's death, which it might itself have hastened or made more agonizing or degrading. And orthodoxy's politicians even wanted to call in the law so as to convert the whole lending-operation into a forced loan, renewable on a perhaps daily basis.

But this was what made many of the heterodox around the 1840s so confident as well as so angry. They interpreted moves for the legal privileging of orthodoxy not simply as short-term threat but as sign of long-term bankruptcy, as a desperately 'un-British' lunge towards absolutist interventionism. True, this perspective could afford to blur or overlook Wakley's struggle to keep the state as no more than the guarantor of his profession.[38] But, viewed at the receiving-end by any of Wakley's 'objects', the distortion is understandable. And such anti-absolutist polemic was to be part of the rhetoric of more than one medical movement during the second half of the century: anti-vaccinationism, for one, or the agitation against the Contagious Diseases Acts.

But by then the heterodox confidence – which, for example, had taken homoeopathic patients and sympathizers in mostly respectable deputation to Whitehall during the 1850s with a demand to be allowed to practise on the troops in the Crimea[39] – was, if not fading, becoming increasingly spasmodic. We can see this waning as not merely 'post-1858' but also as 'post-1840s' and much else. For, in that decade, the fundamental situation often felt more fluid than it was to later. Not that all or even most supporters of one or more heterodox approaches were necessarily political radicals: in this, the position varied. Medical botany may have been unusual in the overwhelming plebeianness of its activists and in the consistency of its democratic epistemology and rhetoric. Homoeopathy, phrenology, mesmerism and phreno-mesmerism, by contrast, seem to have offered an enticing terrain for advocates of the widest possible range of class agendas during the 1830s and 1840s, for ordering and not always for levelling or even modestly shuffling, the social hierarchy.[40] In turn, these agendas sometimes affected strategy for medical reform, but not necessarily.

The point is merely that, when hope or dread of fundamental change is as widespread as it was into the 1840s, institutional change – or here, for the heterodox, liberation – is likelier to seem easy. Obviously, though, the more radically democratic one's politics, the easier the fit with a democratic epistemology – or, at least, the easier one's contempt for élitist or meritocratic epistemologies, let alone for 'old physic', however intimidating its newly reinforced legal status.

Notes

1. Roger Cooter, 'Bones of contention? Orthodox medicine and the mystery of the bonesetters' craft', in W. F. Bynum and Roy Porter (eds), *Medical Fringe and Medical Orthodoxy,* 1750–1850 (London, 1987).
2. J. H. Warner, 'Medical sectarianism, therapeutic conflict and the shaping of orthodox professional identity in antebellum American medicine', in Bynum and Porter (eds), *Medical Fringe and Medical Orthodoxy.*
3. Even though Bynum has talked as if each had its own 'cosmology' (Bynum and Porter, *Medical Fringe and Medical Orthodoxy*, p. 24), it depends what we mean by cosmology.

4. L. Barrow, *Independent Spirits: Spiritualism and English Plebeians, 1850–1910* (London, 1986), particularly ch. 4.

5. Anonymous editorial, *Homoeopathic Record (Medical, Social and Scientific)*, n.s. zx, 2 (1857), 185–7.

6. As by Edward Shorter in conversation during a symposium at the Wellcome Institute, London, July 1983.

7. As was S. T. Hall: see Barrow, *Independent Spirits*, p. 176. See also L. Barrow, 'An imponderable liberator: J. J. Garth Wilkinson', in R. Cooter, *Studies in the History of Alternative Medicine* (London, 1988).

8. Philip A. Nicholl, *Homoeopathy and the Medical Profession* (London, 1988). For Frederic Quin, see Edward Hamilton, M.D., *A Memoir of F. H. F. Quin* (1879). For Spencer T. Hall, see *Memoir of S. T. Hall*, from the *Glasgow Examiner*, October 1884 and numerous works by Hall himself; Barrow (*Independent Spirits: Spiritualism and English Plebeians, 1850–1910*). The self-taught Hall – a travelling showman-mesmerist before he settled down as a hydropath and homoeopath – avoided the normal British qualifications and can thus symbolize the down-market side of homoeopathy as much as Quin can the opposite side.

9. See, e.g., Barrow, *Independent Spirits*, index entries on Elliotson, (or, later, George Wyld).

10. E.g. *Dr Skelton's Botanic Record and Family Herbal*, September, October, November 1852, pp. 79f., 87, 128; March and December 1853, pp. 161f., 311f.; February 1854, pp. 349f.; Barrow, *Independent Spirits*, pp. 185, 188–91; see also P. S. Brown, 'Herbalists and medical botanists in mid 19th century Britain with special reference to Bristol', *Medical History*, 26 (1982); P. S. Brown, 'The vicissitudes of herbalism in late 19th and early 20th century Britain', *Medical History*, 29 (1985); J. F. C. Harrison, 'Early Victorian radicals and the medical fringe', in Bynum and Porter (eds), *Medical Fringe and Medical Orthodoxy*; Ursula Miley and J. V. Pickstone, 'Medical botany around 1850: American medicine in industrial Britain', in Cooter, *Studies in the History of Alternative Medicine*. For Coffin, see Albert I. Coffin *A Botanic Guide to Health and the Natural Pathology of Disease* (with portrait), (Leeds, 1845). The allegedly '36th edition' London, 1866; plus other works.

11. Nicholl, *Homoeopathy and the Medical Profession*. Northampton, *Homoeopathic Record*, March 1856, 71–82.

12. Dorothy Porter and Roy Porter, *Patient's Progress: Doctors and Doctoring in 18th-century England* (Stanford, 1989; Cambridge, 1989), particularly pp. 205f., 208, 214. The broadest and most detailed unravelling of the paradoxes in the eighteenth-century English-British state is surely John Brewer, *The Sinews of Power: War, Money and the English State, 1688–1783* (London, 1989).

13. Gareth Stedman Jones, 'Rethinking Chartism', in *Languages of Class: Studies in English Working-Class History, 1832–1982* (London, 1983).

14. The most elaborate, if occasionally rhetorical, argument for the existence of an Anglo-British 'parliamentary absolutism' – among much else – is Tom Nairn, *The Enchanted Glass: Britain and Its Monarchy* (London 1988).

15. Miley and Pickstone, 'Medical botany around 1850', p. 152.

16. Phil Gardner, *The Lost Elementary Schools of England* (London, 1984).

17. Barrow, *Independent Spirits*; the best way into Wallace remains F. M. Turner, *Between Science and Religion* (London, 1974), ch. 4.

18. Bynum and Porter (eds), *Medical Fringe and Medical Orthodoxy*, preface.

19. Ibid., p. 55n.

20. S. W. F. Holloway, 'The orthodox fringe: the origins of the Pharmaceutical Society of Great Britain', in Bynum and Porter (eds), *Medical Fringe and Medical Orthodoxy*.

21. Roy Porter, 'The patient's view: doing medical history from below', cyclostyled paper, 1987; see Roy Porter, *Health for Sale: Quackery in England, 1660–1850*, (Manchester, 1989); D. and R. Porter, *Patient's Progress*.

22. See particularly Ruth Richardson, *Death, Dissection and the Destitute* (London, 1988).

23. *Lancet*, 21 May 1853, 15 July 1854, 11 November 1854. Wakley's direct authorship of these editorials is not certain, but his indirect or direct influence on their content and style surely stands out.

24. *Lancet*, 15 July 1854, 35.

25. *Lancet*, 21 May 1853, 476.

26. As note 23.

27. Terry Parssinen, 'Professional deviants and the history of medicine: medical mesmerists in Victorian Britain', in Roy Wallis (ed.), *On the Margin of Science: The Social Construction of Rejected Knowledge*, 1979, *Sociological Review*, monograph, p. 111.

28. W. C. Engledue, *Cerebral Physiology and Materialism*, (London, 1842, p10f). Reprinted from the *Medical Times*, but was published by James Watson, a hero of the 'War of the Unstamped', that is of the mass campaign, a decade and more previously, for press freedom. (For Watson, see W. J. Linton *James Watson, a memoir*, Manchester, 1880.)

29. E. g. *Zoist*, 2 (1844–5): 269.

30. *London Medical Gazette*, 23 August 1844, quoted in Parssinen, 'Professional deviants and the history of medicine', p. 109.

31. *Lancet*, 1846, I: 687–91.

32. Robert Darnton, *Mesmerism and the End of the Enlightenment in France* (London: Harvard University Press, 1968).

33. *Lancet*, 1 (1844), 581, 586; *British and Foreign Medical Review*, 8 (1839), 195 (confirmable via *D.N.B.*); *British and Foreign Medical Review*, 24 (1847): postscript, particularly p. 494.

34. L. Barrow, 'A Tale of Two Bladders: the pitfalls of expertise during the climactic decade of British medical reform', article, forthcoming. For a general argument that the spread of physical anaesthetics was surprisingly complicated, see M. Pernick, *Calculus of Suffering* (London: 1987).

35. *Lancet*, 20 June 1846, 687–91.

36. *Lancet*, 20 June 1846, 687–91, emphasis in original.

37. *Lancet*, 20 June 1846, 687–91, emphasis in original.

38. See, e.g., Ivan Waddington, *The Medical Profession in the Industrial Revolution* (London, 1984), particularly p. 78.

39. *Lancet*, 1855, I: 369. The list of petitioners was large and often most prestigious: see Barrow ('A Tale of Two Bladders').

40. Barrow, *Independent Spirits*, pp. 76–84.

8

William Brande and the chemical education of medical students

Elizabeth Haigh

When William Thomas Brande (1788–1866) resigned his position as Professor of Chemistry at the Royal Institution in 1852 after a tenure of nearly four decades, he was apparently well pleased with his achievements in the job. For example, he claimed with justification that his were the first lectures to give 'so extended a view of chemistry, and of its applications'. It was a considerable feat in view of that science's explosive development in the first half of the nineteenth century. In his speech of resignation, he expressed his pride in the fact that he was leaving the Royal Institution 'more prosperous than at any former period; its scientific fame more prevalent; its foundations more secure; its halls more frequented; its usefulness more acknowledged'.[1] The Managers of the Royal Institution gave him credit for this happy state of affairs, putting on record their apparently warmly held conviction that the reputation which the Institution had maintained as a school of chemistry was due to Brande's personal reputation, his scientific achievements, and his assiduous dedication to good teaching.[2]

Indeed, Brande enjoyed a reputation as London's foremost chemist. He had not confined himself to the Royal Institution but had generally participated in London's scientific activity. He was, for example, an original member of the Chemical Society founded in 1841 and a Fellow of the Royal Societies of London and Edinburgh. He accumulated honours from and held membership in a variety of foreign scientific societies as far away as Moscow and New York. Shortly after his resignation, Oxford University made him an Honorary Doctor of Civil Law.[3] His considerable reputation in 1852 is noteworthy when we consider that he is virtually unknown in the history of chemistry today. What is particularly interesting, however, is the observation that, as early as the 1870s, he had virtually vanished from the history of the Royal Institution. It is not simply that an exaggerated reputation had been justifiably cut down to size. For about a century, it was almost as though he had never existed.

Brande had come to the Royal Institution in 1813, succeeding Sir Humphry Davy as Professor of Chemistry. During the ensuing thirty-nine years, he lectured for hundreds of hours in a number of institutions, wrote numerous books and articles, and acted as chemical consultant to government officials, businessmen, merchants, and manufacturers who approached the Royal Institution about a wide variety of problems. During his tenure there, Brande probably did at least as much to guide and to shape the Royal Institution as anyone before or since. As Morris Berman has clearly demonstrated, it was largely because of Brande's work at a crucial time for the Royal Institution that it was transformed from an organization serving largely the interests of the landed gentry into a professionally orientated establishment which popularized science and served a wide range of such public health and commercial interests as preoccupied the professional middle class. Not surprisingly, this coincided with a similar transition from an agrarian to an industrial ethos in society in general. Brande was a relatively new kind of professional, a business-like, practical chemist whose approach to his work was strongly utilitarian. As he saw it, the main value of the sciences was to enhance commerce, education, public health, and human well-being in general – and not least his own reputation! We are familiar with his type today, but, in the pre-Victorian period, the scientific consultant was just emerging to suit the requirements of a growing middle class.[4] While his type would proliferate in ensuing decades, Brande himself was something of a pioneer.

Brande trained as an apothecary and kept medicine always at the centre of his professional life. He began his career at a time when licensing, better education, and improved professional standards for medical practitioners generally were being widely promoted. He took advantage of this to make the Royal Institution a centre for their scientific and especially their chemical education.[5] By forging timely and far-sighted links between medicine and chemistry, he was a major promoter of medical professionalization in the critical first half of the nineteenth century.

Brande was born into a prosperous family of apothecaries who had been attached to the royal household for generations, serving the Hanoverian monarchs both in Hanover and London since the eighteenth century.[6] His father was apothecary to Queen Charlotte and medicines were supplied to King George III from the Brande pharmacy on Arlington Street.[7] Under the circumstances, it would have been difficult for young William not to make something of himself. In 1802, he was apprenticed to his older brother who was a licentiate of the Royal Company of Apothecaries. He studied anatomy at the Windmill Street School made famous by William Hunter, chemistry at St. George's Hospital, and attended some of Sir Humphry Davy's chemistry lectures at the Royal Institution. Indeed, he credited Davy with giving him a taste for chemistry at public lectures he attended, as early as 1801, while still a pupil at Westminster School. By 1805, at the age of 17, Brande was dabbling in that grey area between medicine and chemistry dubbed 'animal chemistry', and publishing papers in *Nicholson's Journal, The Philosophical Transactions*, and other contemporary journals. In 1813, he was awarded the Copley Medal, the Royal Society's highest award, for a paper 'On the state and quantity of alcohol in fermented liquors'. Indisputably a diligent man, Brande was always ambitious, with a nose for success, adept at making the contacts which would best promote his career.

Brande began his lecturing career as early as 1808 when he is said to have delivered two courses of lectures on pharmaceutical chemistry at a private establishment known as Dr. Hooper's Medical Theatre in Burlington Gardens. A year later, he lectured on physics and chemistry at a private 'New Medico-Chemical School' on Windmill Street. He finished his apprenticeship, becoming a full-fledged apothecary, in February 1810. In 1811, Brande was appointed Professor of Chemistry and Materia Medica at the Apothecaries' Company whose members were anxious, 'to give a scientific character to the art'.[8] About the same time, he was hired to lecture on chemical philosophy at the Royal Institution, taking the place of Davy who, having married a wealthy woman, declared he wished to do less teaching. Brande succeeded to Davy's chair in October 1813. Six months later, he proposed to its managers that the Royal

Institution's laboratory be used as a classroom for medical students. They agreed, anticipating that it would bring in much needed income, and Brande moved his class of medical students from Windmill Street and from St. George's Hospital to Albermarle Street. The Royal Institution provided Brande with superb physical facilities and its already considerable reputation as a laboratory and teaching institution.[9] Brande gave it his ambitious drive and industry and a flock of student apothecaries eager for professional respectability. Brande, the Royal Institution, and eventually the students all enjoyed an increase in prestige and income as a result.

The timing was good. Brande began his professional career just as the modern structure of medical education began to emerge in England. Until the Medical Act of 1858 merged practitioners of medicine into a single profession, there were basically three kinds of doctors – physicians, surgeons, and apothecaries. The learned, university-trained physicians were the gentlemen of the medical professions, cultured and educated, but often with little or no hospital or practical experience. Newman reports that, as late as 1834, a Cambridge MA could take an MD without attending any lectures on medicine, without any hospital practice, or without even an examination. He could then practise without being licensed. It was up to him whether or not he would listen to lectures and 'walk the wards' for practical experience. The physicians' clientele tended to be wealthy but, by the nineteenth century, physicians were losing ground to surgeons and apothecaries. The craftsmanlike surgeons, besides operating, were allowed to treat patients with externally applied salves or lotions. Again, there were no legally required qualifications, but it was usual for a surgeon to start with a five-year apprenticeship and, from 1813 at least, to add a year's attendance at the surgical practice in a hospital. Surgeons had a professional organization in the Royal College of Surgeons. The apothecaries, originally shopkeepers, largely learned their trade simply by serving an apprenticeship. Increasingly, as apothecaries gradually acquired more status and organization, persons held dual qualifications as surgeon-apothecaries. These more or less official groups shared the business of dispensing nostrums and services with midwives, herbalists, druggists, galvanizers, and a multitude of quacks.

Increasingly, apothecaries were becoming the medical advisers to the growing middle class and even to the upper classes. It is estimated that, in London in 1800, there were some twenty apothecaries for every physician. Outside the city, there were practically no physicians at all. The Oxford- and Cambridge-trained members of the College of Physicians, therefore, were gradually becoming almost irrelevant to medicine. In spite of the fact that few regulations governed the establishment of any sort of medical practice, medical education was increasingly being promoted by various private schools. It was becoming customary for students to attend some lectures on their own initiative and to acquire some hospital experience before establishing themselves as practitioners.[10]

The Apothecaries' Act of 1815 was the first attempt to control this group's medical practice officially. It established a Court of Examiners to evaluate the competence of all future apothecaries, although it did not interfere with those already practising. It required that all future practitioners be licensed only after examination by the Apothecaries' Company at the end of a five-year apprenticeship. (For medical education and the Apothecaries' Act, see the chapter by Susan Lawrence in this volume.) An aspiring apothecary would have to demonstrate that he had taken lessons in chemistry, materia medica, anatomy, medicine, physiology, and botany, and that he had practised six months in a hospital, infirmary, or dispensary. By the 1840s, five out of every six of the students in London hospitals were working for an apothecary's licence. So it was that the Act entrusted the Society of Apothecaries with responsibility for the great majority of the medical practitioners of England and Wales.[11]

The case for the other requirements in the apothecaries' curriculum seems clear enough, but it is interesting to speculate why it was judged necessary for physicians to learn botany and chemistry. Course outlines demonstrate that their contents went far beyond the therapeutic properties of certain plants or chemicals. Science was built into the apothecaries' curriculum largely because, to be respectable in the nineteenth century, medicine had to be seen to be a scientifically rooted profession and apothecaries to be learned men. Scientific theory, of course, contributed little to the practice of medicine. Science, nevertheless, loomed very large in the eyes of medical reformers, presumably because it teaches an outlook on reality and a methodology which were deemed appropriate for a modern physician. It was the scientific outlook which distinguished him from the quack and from varieties of do-it-yourselfer. This point was made, for example, in the *Lancet* in 1824 where one reads that there is 'not a more important or valuable branch of Medical education than chemistry . . . now justly regarded as the ground-work of all medical knowledge'.[12] The seventeenth-century apothecary had been a tradesman dispensing advice with the nostrums he sold in his shop. By 1815, he was starting the final process of an evolution which would transform him into a scientific, professional member of a self-regulating company. Brande was an instrument of that evolution. His lectures to medical students incorporated something of physics, of vegetable chemistry, of animal chemistry, and of geology, all with a view to making the physician a man of learning. Presumably that is still our purpose in requiring much of the science of our pre-medical curricula.

The extension of the audience for a scientific education contributed to making the lofty and exclusive status of physicians shakier. Hitherto, they alone among medical practitioners could lay claim to any particular learning or refinement. But now apothecaries were appropriating learning and anticipating a scientific future. Accordingly, chemistry was a powerful ideological lever which allowed the apothecary to become the professional and the medical man in the form of the general practitioner.

There is, however, another facet to this. Anatomy and physiology obviously help one to understand the nature of the body. By 1800, it began to look as though chemistry might do the same. The faith of the old iatrochemists was re-emerging in modern dress. Accordingly, 'vegetable chemistry' and 'animal chemistry' were substantial components of Brande's chemistry textbooks and lectures. Merely embryonic studies when he began his career, they were shortly to develop into organic chemistry and, especially, biochemistry. Their origins in the nineteenth century go back to the work of scientists who were often physicians first. Like them, Brande came to chemistry, apparently the study which best suited his nature, from medical studies.

In Britain, animal chemistry had received great stimulus from the work of such persons as Joseph Black, whose investigations on specific heat Brande seemed particularly to admire; from Joseph Priestley, who did important work on oxygen and carbonic acid – the 'goodness of air'; and from Henry

Cavendish who discovered hydrogen and the composition of water. While discoveries about the nature of heat and gases were suggestive for the investigation of living nature, probably the most dramatic application of chemistry to physiology had been Antoine Lavoisier's and Pierre Laplace's demonstration, late in the eighteenth century, of the equation between respiration and combustion. In any case, by 1800, chemical studies had finally progressed to the point where they could begin to throw significant light on organic processes. The animal chemists, therefore, could build on foundations unavailable to the iatrochemists. The timing was just right for Brande.

The very first course in animal chemistry seems to have been offered at the Lycée in Paris in 1790 by the physician and chemist Antoine Fourcroy who emphasized the relations between chemistry and natural history and their application to medicine. He studied many solids and fluids in the animal body in sickness and in health.[14] Animal and vegetable chemistry grew rapidly after 1800. The first book devoted to *Animal Chemistry*, one which included many analyses of animal tissues and fluids, was published in 1806 by the vitalist Jons Jacob Berzelius, a Swedish physician-turned-chemist who gave us the words 'isomerism' and 'protein'. Largely interested in inorganic chemistry, he laboured hard to demonstrate his conviction that the laws of chemical combination held in the organic world. In doing so, he was to work out the formulae of many organic substances such as starch, sugar, citric acid, tartaric acid, and so on.[15] Developing techniques of quantitative organic analysis about 1810, Joseph Louis Gay-Lussac demonstrated conclusively that carbon, hydrogen, oxygen, and nitrogen are the primary constituents of all organic compounds.[16] Deriving from that was the very significant work of Justus von Liebig on nutrition in which he attempted to deduce the actual chemical transformations which the three classes of nutrients undergo in the body. These are, of course, but a fraction of an increasingly large number of persons who framed their questions about living nature in chemical terms. Grounded on such foundations, animal chemistry would quickly evolve into organic chemistry and finally biochemistry, the special chemistry of living nature, with its particular assumptions, techniques, and even language.

Brande participated in this burgeoning application of chemistry to physiology. His earliest paper, published in 1805 when he was only 17 years old, was on the subject of benzoin, a gum resin used in perfumes and medicines.[17] He was given the project by Charles Hatchett, an analyst and mineralogist who had his own laboratory in which he allowed Brande to work while he was still an apprentice.[18] In the next few years. Brande would go on to investigate the theory of respiration, urinary calculi, the invertebral fluid of fishes and invertebrates, albumen, fermentation, blood, and many other topics. Over the years, in his capacity as chief chemist at the Royal Institution, he would also undertake much work in inorganic chemistry, largely as he received commissions to do so. He was, for example, the Superintendent of Machinery and Clerk of the Irons in the Mint from 1825, a lucrative position he received after investigating some questions having to do with the quality of metals in coinage. Left to himself, however, one gets the impression that he remained a medical man, straying towards questions relating one way or another to living nature or to public health.

Brande's youthful acquaintance with Hatchett was fortuitous. The older man was a manager of the Royal Institution, which almost certainly accounts for Brande's appointments there in 1811 and 1813. In 1818, Brande married Hatchett's daughter. He appears to have had an instinct for useful contacts. For example, while a student at St. George's Hospital, Brande attracted the favourable attention of the influential surgeon Everard Home. Brande's fellow student at St. George's was Benjamin Collins Brodie who was destined to become a leader of the London medical profession. In the future, Brodie was to undertake distinguished work on the nervous system, examining its effect on the heart, on the production of animal heat, and on the control of gastric secretions.[19] In their student days, under Home's direction, Brande and Brodie were to work together on various problems in animal chemistry.

The point is that in October 1808, with a group of fellows of the Royal Society including Hatchett, Davy, Home, and Brodie, Brande was a founding member of a Society for the Promotion of Animal Chemistry which was placed under the protection of the Royal Society. For years, the group met four times annually at the home of Hatchett or Home; Brande, probably the youngest member, served as its secretary.[20] The Society seems gradually to have faded away, its concerns giving way to new areas of investigation and research.

In spite of a fair amount of this sort of more or less private scientific teaching and association, there was little formal education in science available in England early in the nineteenth century. In 1830, Charles Babbage deplored the Government's neglect of science and the fact that, unlike in Prussia or elsewhere, one could not pursue a scientific field as a profession in England. There were so few lucrative possibilities in industry or the universities, he argued, that one needed a private fortune to be able to study it at all.[21] This official neglect of science goes a long way towards explaining why the lectures of Davy, his undeniably appealing style notwithstanding, were so popular in the early years of the Royal Institution, and why Brande, Faraday, Young, and other lecturers in the Royal Institution and elsewhere continued to attract hundreds of formal and informal students for many decades into the nineteenth century.[22]

It was largely due to Brande's diligence that the Royal Institution acquired a reputation as a school of chemistry at the very time that the medical profession began to emphasize scientific education. Brande's chemistry lectures were given three times a week from October to April of each year, a total of some eighty lectures annually. Up to 120 students paid Brande four guineas each for the privilege of enrolling. He turned one third of the money over to the Royal Institution as a kind of rent for the use of their premises. All this was, of course, in addition to the Royal Institution's numerous public lectures, on a great variety of subjects, many of which Brande also delivered.

By the 1840s, attendance at the chemistry courses declined dramatically as hospitals increasingly began to provide their own lecturers and teaching facilities. This, however, was compensated for by a growing demand in the city for laboratory facilities to train people to do research and analyses. As chemical discoveries prodigiously expanded, chemistry was seen to be relevant in more and more areas. For example, the chemists and druggists formed their own Pharmaceutical Society in 1841. A year later, they created the first School of Pharmacy. It required, of course, laboratory instruction. With an eye to fulfilling a demand, Brande, supported by Faraday, brought a proposal to the Royal Institution Board of Managers for the creation of a School of Practical Chemistry to train research chemists and of a separate laboratory elsewhere to undertake analyses on a commercial basis. This would have displaced the School of Chemistry for medical students. After expressing interest initially, however, the managers turned down the proposal on the grounds that there was not sufficient space.[23] If that was merely an excuse, one guess is that they feared that it would become a financial liability. Another is that it was the result of a growing tendency to downgrade the Royal Institution's professional teaching functions. Accordingly, it gradually drifted towards making research its primary objective. It was after that that Michael Faraday came into his own, producing the splendidly innovative work which made his such a distinguished career of discovery. In the 1860s, when Henry Bence Jones was Secretary of the Royal Institution, research was officially pronounced to be its first and essential objective.[24] As we shall see, Bence Jones preferred to forget that it had ever been anything else in spite of the fact that he had personally attended chemistry lectures at the Royal Institution while a medical student enrolled at St. George's Hospital.

It may be instructive to look at the chemical instruction which Brande offered his medical students. An extant set of student's lecture notes from 1812 show us that, from the beginning, Brande offered a concise statement of the current state of chemical knowledge. As the field rapidly developed, so did the scope of his lectures and books. Early on, in 1812, he divided chemistry into *synthetic* and *analytic* categories, the first proceeding from simple to complex bodies and the latter breaking compounds down into their component parts. It was a scientific methodology emphasized by the French ideologists and enjoying a great vogue early in the nineteenth century. In that early work, Brande went on to consider heat, light (particles emanating from luminous bodies), and some fifty *simple* or elemental natural bodies. He dealt with the chemistry of oxygen, chlorine, water, nitrogen, atmospheric air, coal, gas, and certain acids. It would seem to be as up-to-date a course as one could reasonably expect to have had at the time.

From 1816 onwards, the *Quarterly Journal of Science & Art* offered a prospectus of Brande's courses. Almost certainly without his permission, although the publicity would not have displeased him, his lectures from 1827–8 were reproduced in the *Lancet* along with those of other persons who lectured to medical students on various subjects. It was part of the editor Thomas Wakley's belligerent campaign to reform the medical profession and to make it, as he saw it, less self-serving.[25]

But the most complete work available to students was Brande's textbook, the *Manual of Chemistry*. The first edition of 1819 was sensibly dedicated to his father-in-law. The massive work was to go through six editions and be treated for decades as *the* contemporary chemistry textbook. It came to be translated into French, German, and Italian, giving Brande a European reputation.[26] He tended to start his books and lectures with a substantial historical introduction, on one occasion looking at least as far back as Tubal Caine.[27] The roots of modern chemistry he took to be the work of Bacon, Boyle, Hooke, and Newton, upon whom such eminent pioneers as Black and Lavoisier modelled themselves. He began the 1819 exposition by considering the 'powers' connected with chemical change – attraction, heat, electricity, and light. He treated combustion at length. By then, he was demonstrating a cursory knowledge of atomic theory and speculating on the mechanics of reactions. This broad-ranging discussion was followed by substantial sections on animal chemistry, vegetable chemistry, and geology.

The third edition incorporated some of Faraday's work in an enlarged section on electricity. Geology was dropped, probably because it was developing its own language and theory faster than Brande could keep up with it. By the fourth edition, enriched with some 200 illustrations, Brande began to use Whewell's chemical symbols. The final edition of 1848, described as 'one of the best chemistry books in the first half of the nineteenth century', showed equations. As chemistry continued to develop at an accelerating pace, Brande incorporated whatever was new, writing eventually with ease about such specialized subjects as crystallization, dimorphism, chemical affinity, equivalent weights and volumes, and spectral analysis. Throughout it all, he never lost his eye for things practical, the utilitarian in him staying alert to the social, technological, and commercial applications which gave coherence and purpose to it all.[28]

In the meantime, Brande was also delivering regular lecture courses in pharmacy at the Apothecaries' Hall. Between 1825 and 1833, he published three editions of a *Manual of Pharmacy*, a reference book which outlined the occurrence, preparation, dosage, and effects of drugs sanctioned by the Royal College of Pharmacy of London. It became a standard handbook for nineteenth-century pharmacists. Besides these works, he edited a *Dictionary of Materia Medica* in 1839 and a *Dictionary of Science & Art* in 1842, a 1343-page general encyclopaedia which was to appear in six editions.[29] It addressed a wide range of subjects from architecture, through the various sciences, law, general, literature, and even theology.

The scope of Brande's work can be seen by even a cursory glance at the *Quarterly Journal of Science & Art*, published by the Royal Institution between 1816 and 1831. It was initially his idea that the Royal Institution publicize its work with a journal. He edited it and was largely responsible for its contents which reflected his bias towards medicinal and industrial chemistry. It turned out to be a kind of trade journal whose secondary purpose was to co-ordinate professional information. That is to say, in addition to publishing research articles, it reviewed the latest books, made announcements, and generally kept the technical reader up to date on the most recent developments in many fields.[30] With the *Lancet*, it was one of the first modern journals to serve an emerging professional group. It reinforces my claim on behalf of Brande as a promoter of medical professionalization, and it contributed to the Royal Institution's prestige and income.

Brande offered to resign from his lectures in 1846 so the position could go to a 'younger, more active and renowned person'. The managers declined his offer, reluctant to lose the man who had made their Institution the leading school of chemistry in England.[31] Besides, St. George's Hospital at least still wanted the courses continued. Brande finally left the job six years later to take up a lucrative position as Chief Officer of the Coinage Department of the Royal Mint, where he had been living and working part-time for some twenty-seven years already.

About that same time Brande also resigned from the Apothecaries' Hall. As with the Royal Institution, there were many expressions of goodwill on both sides. The apothecaries in particular treated him as an honoured member of their company for they hung his portrait among those of a mere handful of other worthies, and they named a laboratory and the 'Brande Rooms' after him.[32]

In most histories of chemistry, Brande gets passing mention as a teacher and as something of a pioneer in animal chemistry. That is probably appropriate for it would be hard to defend him as a particularly innovative chemist. What is remarkable, however, is his virtual disappearance from histories of the Royal Institution and that within a mere five years of his death. Bence Jones's book on *The Royal Institution; its Founder & First Professors* ignored him completely, an extraordinary and churlish omission.[33] So did Sir Henry Holland who described his own connections in the Royal Institution as invaluable, naming Faraday, Young, and Davy who 'kept me in the train of those great discoveries which have illustrated their names and given a well-merited fame to the place in which they were made'.[34] An 1872 biography of *Michael Faraday* by one J. J. Gladstone mentions Brande merely to remark that Faraday prepared Brande's apparatus for his lectures 'and helped him to produce the strange transformations of the chemical art',[35] implying that Brande would have had difficulty managing them on his own. Brande was even absent from an 1875 article written about the chemistry laboratories at the Royal Institution.[36] A laboratory constructed there in 1896 was named the Davy-Faraday lab. To have disparaged Brande the man, Brande the chemist, or Brande the teacher as deficient in one way or another might have been defensible. To make him disappear is the most eloquent put-down of all.

This pointed ungenerosity on the part of his students and younger contemporaries, of course, distorted the history of the Royal Institution and its laboratories. There is a good possibility that there was something personal in it. Having been something of a self-promoter, Brande had undoubtedly created resentment. It probably also has to do with the image and the purpose of the Royal Institution as certain members perceived it. Brande acted as if he believed the Royal Institution's proper function was to teach science and to popularize it and to make it the handmaiden of commerce, business, and technology. For Bence Jones and Spottiswoode, the Institution was properly the home of great research.[37] And they were prepared to ignore the reality of many years for the sake of that image. Brande the teacher and business-like consultant could be dismissed as merely an anomaly. Davy and Faraday had also been required to do routine, journeyman analyses, answering questions about copper sheathing on ships, agricultural practices, coal-gas lighting, leather tanning, and what have you.[38] But it is for other reasons that they became the subjects of biographies. Brande never ventured far beyond answering limited and practical questions. Accordingly, he never made discoveries anywhere near as important as those of Davy and Faraday.

The neglect of Brande persisted into the present century. In 1901, another biographer of Faraday would have it that he had saved the Institution from ruin, a condition presumably created by Brande although his name is not mentioned. While Silvanus praised the very high standards of the Institution's lectures which had long drawn fashionable crowds, he referred to Brande only to dismiss him as a 'humdrum lecturer, not exactly an inspiring person'.[39]

As recently as the 1960s, L. Pearce Williams scarcely mentioned Brande in his works on Faraday and he certainly gave him no credit at all for influencing Faraday's career in spite of their long association.[40] Finally, in the 1970s, two theses looked seriously at his contributions to chemistry and its teaching.[41] Then in 1978, in Berman's fine study of the Royal Institution, there was an acknowledgement of Brande's considerable contribution to shaping the Royal Institution and to keeping it solvent and relevant to nineteenth-century needs. Berman disparaged him, nevertheless, as 'the scientific version of the Dickensian Gradgrind'.[42]

As science came to be studied by ever increasing numbers of people in the nineteenth century, and as it came to be more and more widely applied, the number of Gradgrinds emerging from our technical schools and universities also continued to grow. By far the majority of today's scientists would have to be dismissed as such if we applied any sort of tests of originality and creativity to their achievements. That is, of course, the consequence of creating a profession and of making it accessible to large numbers of people. It was his very Gradgrind qualities which made Brande a pioneer in the promotion of a broadly based scientific outlook, for he understood that the medical future belonged to scientifically orientated men. He taught his students much about the nature of basic science, he promoted professional publishing, and he generally participated in the creation of the modern physician. Throughout his professional life, he treated science as an essential component of contemporary technological and commercial activity. As a chemical consultant motivated by things practical, he participated in western Europe's extraordinary industrial revolution which was to continue to absorb increasing numbers of his type of thorough, dedicated, and versatile, albeit not particularly creative, Gradgrinds.

Notes

1. 'Resignation of Professor Brande', *Rev. John Barlow Scrapbook, RI Archives,* Box 150, p. 33. See also the 'Letter of W. T. Brande to Benjamin Brodie', 7 November 1849, *RI Archives,* IX, 122E. He wrote to Brodie as follows:

> It has always appeared to me, and in recent innovations I have seen nothing to shake my opinion that the main objects of the Royal Institution are not to teach the minutiae of practical chemistry to persons who are following it professionally, or in detail, but to diffuse a general taste for the science; to give, in the theatre, that kind of Chemical Instruction, which without in any way compromising the high character of the Institution, shall aim rather at generalities than at particulars, that is, shall not be unacceptable to those who rank highest in the Science, and shall at the same time interest their opposites.

2. Quoted by A. S. Forgan, 'The Royal Institution of Great Britain, 1840–1873', thesis submitted for the degree of PhD, 1977, pp. 64–5. Taken from *Managers' Minutes,* IX, 417 (16 November 1846).

3. Aubrey A. Tulley, 'The chemical studies of William Thomas Brande, 1788–1866', MSc thesis, University of London, 1970, pp. 40–1.

4. Morris Berman, 'Introduction', *The Archives of the Royal Institution of Great Britain in facsimile: Minutes of the Managers' Meetings, 1799–1900* (London: Scolar Press, 1973), vol. VI, pp. ii–vi. Also Morris Berman, *Social Change and Scientific Organization: The Royal Institution, 1799–1844* (London: Heinemann, 1978), ch. 4, pp. 100–55.

5. Berman, 'Introduction', *The Archives of the Royal Institution,* vol. VI, pp. iii–vi.

6. For biographical details, see Berman, *Social Change and Scientific Organization,* pp. 130–55; Donovan Chilton and Noel J. Coley, 'The laboratories of the Royal Institution in the nineteenth century', *Ambix,* 27, 3 (1980): 173–203; Edward Ironmonger, 'Forgotten worthies of the Royal Institution. (1) William Thomas Brande (1788–1866)', *Proceedings of the Royal Institution,* 38 (1961): 450–61; Edward Ironmonger, 'Further thoughts on W. T. Brande', *Proceedings of the Royal Institution,* 44 (1970): 262–73; C. H. Spiers, 'William Thomas Brande, leather expert', *Annals of Science,* 25 (1969): 179–201; and Tulley.

7. George Edward Trease, *Pharmacy in History* (London: Baillière, Tindall & Cox, 1964).

8. *Lancet,* 11 January 1824, 57. Quoted by Berman, *Social Change and Scientific Organization,* p. 104.

9. Forgan, 'The Royal Institution', especially ch. 3, pp. 122–68; Berman, 'Introduction', *The Archives of the Royal Institution.*

10. Charles Newman, *The Evolution of Medical Education in the Nineteenth Century* (London: Oxford University Press, 1957); S. W. F. Holloway, 'Medical education in England, 1830–1858', *History,* 49 (1964): 299–324; Stephen Paget, *Memoirs and Letters of Sir James Paget*

(London, 1903), p. 19, for the student's viewpoint; Leslie G. Matthews, *History of Pharmacy in Britain* (Edinburgh and London: Livingstone, 1962); R. H. Shryock, *The Development of Modern Medicine* (New York: Hafner, 1969); R. H. Shryock, 'Nineteenth century medicine', *Journal of World History*, 3 (1957) and 5 (1959); and Trease, *Pharmacy in History*.

11. W. S. C. Copeman, *The Worshipful Society of Apothecaries, London 1617–1967* (London: Pergamon Press, 1967); William Lawrence Burn, *The Age of Equipoise* (London: Allen & Unwin, 1964), pp. 202–11; Bernice Hamilton, 'Medical professions in the eighteenth century', *Economic History Review*, 4 (1951): 163–9; S.W.F. Holloway, 'The Apothecaries' Act, 1815', *Medical History*, 1966: 107–29 and 221–36; Phillip R.C. Elliot, *The Sociology of the Professions* (London: Macmillan, 1972).

12. *Lancet*, 18 March 1824, 384. Quoted by Berman, *Social Change and Scientific Organization*, p. 104.

13. Forgan, 'The Royal Institution', pp. 122–68; and Arnold Chaplin, *Medicine in England during the Reign of George III* (London: Henry Kimpton, 1912).

14. 'Antoine Fourcroy', *Dictionary of Scientific Biography*; J.R. Partington, *A Short History of Chemistry* (London: Macmillan, 1937), esp. ch. 10.

15. 'Jons Jacob Berzelius', *Dictionary of Scientific Biography*; J.R. Partington, *A Short History of Chemistry*, pp. 194–208.

16. J. R. Partington, *A Short History of Chemistry*, ch. 10.

17. W. T. Brande, 'Analytic experiments and observations on benzoin', *Nicholson's Journal*, 10 (1805): 82.

18. W. T. Brande, 'Chemical experiments on Guaiacum', *Philosophical Transactions*, 96 (1806): 89–98. Other works in animal chemistry are discussed in Tulley, 'The chemical studies of William Thomas Brande', pp. 86–159; A. J. Horne, 'A bibliography of William Thomas Brande' (1955), at the Royal Institution, and other biographical accounts.

19. Benjamin Collins Brodie, *Dictionary of Scientific Biography*. After 1840, Brande would teach with Brodie. See Forgan, *The Royal Institution*, p. 140.

20. Tulley, 'The chemical studies of William Thomas Brande', pp. 89–93; Spiers, 'William Thomas Brande', p. 188; Ironmonger, 'Further thoughts'.

21. Charles Babbage, *Reflections on the Decline of Science in England and on some of its Causes* (London: Fellowes, 1830).

22. J. M. Hays, 'The London lecturing empire, 1800–1850', in Ian Inkster and Jack Morell (eds), *Metropolis and Province: Science in British Culture, 1780–1850* (London: Hutchinson, 1983), pp. 91–119; and J. M. Hays, 'Science in the City; the London Institution, 1819–40', *British Journal of the History of Science*, 7 (1974): 146–62; Bernard H. Becker, *Scientific London* (London: Henry S. King, 1874); Edward Ironmonger, 'The Royal Institution and the teaching of science in the nineteenth century', *Proceedings of the Royal Institution*, 37 (1958): 139–58.

23. Sophie Forgan, 'Introduction', *The Archives of the Royal Institution of Great Britain in Facsimile: Minutes of the Managers' Meetings*,

1799–1900 (London: Scolar Press, 1973), vol. IX (December 1837 to April 1847), pp. iii–vi.

24. Forgan, 'The Royal Institution', pp. 137ff.

25. Sir Squire Sprigge, *Life and Times of Thomas Wakley,* (London, 1899); Newman, *The Evolution of Medical Education,* pp. 140–9. Brande contributed an extensive article on 'Chemistry' to the *Encyclopedia Britannica,* supplement to the 4th, 5th, and 6th editions (Edinburgh: Archibald Constable & Co., 1842), vol. III.

26. Tulley, 'The chemical studies of William Thomas Brande', pp. 38–40 and p. 167.

27. Brande, 'Chemistry' Encyclopedia Britannica.

28. Tulley, 'The chemical studies of William Thomas Brande', p. 167.

29. Ibid., pp. 74–5; A. J. Horne, 'A bibliography of William Thomas Brande'.

30. Berman, 'Introduction', vol. VI; Berman, *Social Change and Scientific Organization,* p. 141; Tulley, 'The chemical studies of William Thomas Brande', p. 26.

31. Tulley, 'The chemical studies of William Thomas Brande', p. 35; Ironmonger, 'Further thoughts'.

32. Copeman, *The Worshipful Society of Apothecaries,* p. 90; C. R. B. Barrett, *History of the Society of Apothecaries of London* (London, 1905), pp. 249–251, p. 278.

33. Henry Bence Jones, *The Royal Institution: Its Founder and its First Professors* (London: Longmans, Green & Co., 1871). Also, Henry Bence Jones, *The Life and Letters of Faraday,* 2 vols (London: Longmans, Green & Co., 1870), makes only a cursory reference to Brande's *Manual.*

34. Sir Henry Holland, *Recollections of Past Life* (London: 1872). Also true of George E. Ellis, *Memoir of Sir Benjamin Thomas, Count Rumford.* These and Bence Jones's book *The Royal Institution: Its Founder and its First Professors* are reviewed in 'Royal Institution', *Edinburgh Review,* 135 (1872): 321–46.

35. J. H. Gladstone, *Michael Faraday* (London: Macmillan & Co., 1872).

36. William Spottiswoode, 'On the old and new laboratories at the Royal Institution', *Proceedings of the Royal Institution,* 7 (1873–5): 1–10.

37. Forgan, 'The Royal Institution', p. 285.

38. Berman, 'Introduction'; see especially vol. IV, pp. v–viii.

39. Phillips Thompson Silvanus, *Michael Faraday* (London: Cassell & Co., 1901). See also Sir William A. Tilden, *Famous Chemists* (London: 1930).

40. L. Pearce Williams, 'Michael Faraday's education in science', *Isis,* 51 (1960): 515–30; and L. Pearce Williams, *Michael Faraday: A Biography* (London: Chapman & Hall, 1965).

41. Forgan, 'The Royal Institution', and Tulley, 'The chemical studies of William Thomas Brande'.

42. Berman, *Social Change and Scientific Organization,* p. 132. Spiers, *William Thomas Brande,* describes him as 'dull but competent', p. 191. There are numerous similar examples.

9

A scientific profession: medical reform and forensic medicine in British periodicals of the early nineteenth century

Catherine Crawford

In August 1829 the Society of Apothecaries passed a resolution enjoining candidates for its licence to apply themselves to the study of forensic medicine. The following year, the Society went further and made formal training in the subject a prerequisite for its examination.[1] This enactment was a major event from the perspective of the fledgling medical science referred to variously as medical jurisprudence, legal medicine, or forensic medicine. Most medical students in London at this time sought accreditation by both the College of Surgeons and the Society of Apothecaries, and the latter corporation was examining between 400 and 450 candidates every year.[2] By obliging these people to attend courses of lectures on forensic medicine, the Apothecaries' regulation established the field in medical education and guaranteed teachers of the subject a sizeable, fee-paying audience. Looking back in 1830 on the resolution that had recognized legal medicine the preceding year, the editor of the *London Medical and Surgical Journal* assigned the credit to medical journalism. The Apothecaries' action, he remarked, 'was effected by the independent medical press, which by the bye is of very recent growth amongst us'.[3]

The enthusiasm for the new field evinced by the medical periodicals of the 1810s and 1820s is striking. The *London Medical and Physical Journal* began expressing concern about the paucity of English works on legal medicine in 1809.[4] In 1814 the first issue of the *London Medical Repository* singled out medical jurisprudence in its opening statement, lamenting the neglect of the subject and declaring that the new journal would be giving special attention to this 'important branch of research'. The editors solicited contributions from readers, noting that

'*Medicina Forensis* has yet so little been attended to in this country, that an ample and productive field is left nearly unappropriated'.[5] Between 1814 and 1830, trial reports, articles, notes, and long expository reviews on medico-legal matters appeared frequently in the leading medical journals.[6] These texts were often accompanied by editorial commentary which strenuously asserted the importance of forensic medicine. In fact, the enthusiasm of journal editors to promote the new science tended to outstrip the availability of material. Early in 1818, for example, a subsection headed 'Medical jurisprudence' in the annual 'Retrospect of the progress of medical Science' of the *Medical Repository* began with the editors' expression of regret 'that we have little to notice on this very important division of our Report'. Later that year they made unfavourable comparisons with France and Germany, wishing 'that any thing we could say might impress upon the minds of our countrymen the importance of the study'.[7] In 1824, the editors introduced a regular section on 'Political Medicine' – largely forensic – and declared that the innovation was demanded by the 'great importance, nay necessity' of developing this branch of medicine. They proposed 'to exceed our former labours in regard to forensic medicine' and to offer an article on medico-legal subjects 'every month, if possible; conveying our own sense of their importance, and (we trust) enlarging that of the Profession'.[8]

Active promotion was not limited to the *Medical Repository*; other journals also tended to portray this minor and atypical area of medical practice as central to the concerns of the profession.[9] The visibility of the topic in the medical press was such that, when the medical curriculum was revised at Edinburgh in 1825, Robert Christison argued successfully for the inclusion of medical jurisprudence as an option by pointing to the 'large share of attention it had been experiencing for some time in the British medical journals'.[10]

Why were journal editors so interested in forensic medicine? The arguments and rhetoric by which they promoted the field suggest that forensic medicine had special significance in relation to editors' broader concerns. The medical periodicals of this period shared a commitment to improving the state of medicine as a profession and as a body of knowledge. They sought to make the medical art more objective and certain, to raise standards of education, and to secure legislation that would regulate medical practice more effectively and justly. The early nineteenth century was a period of sustained agitation for reform of this kind, in which the medical press played a self-consciously central role. Though the specific targets of reformist zeal varied, as did the degree of radicalism of the solutions proposed, there was nevertheless broad agreement that the medical world was in need of improvement and that publicity of the kind the weekly and monthly medical press could provide had an important part to play in the process. In this context the subject of forensic medicine acquired a peculiar interest, for it seemed highly relevant to the goals and strategies of medical reformers.

Forensic medicine as exemplar of ideals

An underlying concern of much programmatic medical writing of the late eighteenth and early nineteenth centuries was the problem of medical uncertainty. Medical authors frequently explained that the complexity of the bodily economy and the difficulty of assessing causation made it easy for charlatans to deceive the public with false or exaggerated claims. This pre-occupation with fraud in the form of quackery was accompanied by concern about the prevalance of error in medicine generally. Growing dissatisfaction was expressed in medical journals about the quality of the evidence on which medical knowledge was based.[11] The need for systematic and comprehensive induction was frequently reiterated. Reliance on medical authorities and on analogical reasoning was disapproved of, and it was becoming unacceptable to justify opinions with vague references to personal 'experience'. Scepticism with respect to medical facts was tirelessly preached in the medical press, and there was considerable discussion about methods of obviating inaccuracy and bias in clinical and experimental reports. In 1812 the editors of the *Medical and Physical Journal* apologized for harping on this theme, declaring that duty required them continually to repeat that 'medical opinions are valuable only when founded on incontrovertible facts'.[12] Gilbert Blane's treatise on medical proof, excerpted at length in this journal in 1819, explained that, because medicine was 'an art beset with every species of fallacy, it is of the utmost importance that those who engage in it, should be fully aware of this, and that they should . . . discipline their minds, by a knowledge of the laws of evidence'.[13] An enthusiastic review of Daniel Pring's work on physiology in 1820 was prefaced by a discourse about the necessity of following 'precise rules for distinguishing correct from incorrect reasoning' and 'established facts from probabilities', and for 'determining precisely the progress of a series of successive causation'. Not least among the achievements of Pring's book, according to this reviewer, was the fact that it revealed how weak the evidentiary basis of many established opinions was.[14]

Solutions were sought to the perceived tendency of medical men to disagree on even simple factual questions.[15] It was often pointed out that practitioners lacked objectivity with respect to their own opinions, and proposals were occasionally made for routinely submitting medical disputes to boards of independent assessors. An article on the 'Verification of medical experience' published in 1830 declared that practitioners were lax about evidence because they had little expectation that their facts would be subjected to close scrutiny. What was needed, according to the author, was 'some form of security against the results of careless, unconsidered, and partial observation and experiment being represented as legitimate and undoubted matters of fact'. He proposed that a 'court of inquiry' be instituted to settle contentious points – one that was 'so constituted as to preclude the possibility of personal bias'. Practitioners would observe and analyse more carefully, he commented, 'if they were aware that their assertions . . . would have to abide the test of a prompt and unobjectionable investigation'.[16]

The medical journals themselves functioned as a sort of professional tribunal, providing critical reviews and a forum for debate, and imposing rules on the process of evaluation. For example, the editors of the *Edinburgh Medical and Surgical Journal* explained in 1814 that they would not review a publication by the eye specialist Sir William Adams, in which the success of his operations for cataract was related, because he kept his method a secret. They declared that they would fear some mistake or deception until Adams described his procedure and enabled them to judge the merits of the operation 'scientifically'. This despite the fact that the directors of the Royal Hospital for Seamen had commissioned and monitored the trials, and Adams's success had resulted in a knighthood. Such trappings of authority did not entitle Adams to consideration by the profession, for, the editors remarked, 'it is the *operation* and not the *operator* we look to'.[17] It was repeatedly declared in medical periodicals that unless contributors laid all their cards on the table, so that their conclusions could be fully inquired into by others, medicine could not escape the mire of error and uncertainty which had impeded its progress for so long.

There are obvious resemblances between these demands for rigorous medical proof and the pressures that were exerted on testimony in a court of law. Legal procedures for minimizing doubt in the early nineteenth century included sustained cross-examination, in which evidence and reasoning were challenged by professional advocates who sought to impeach witnesses on grounds of imprecision, inconsistency, and bias. There were also more specific parallels, such as the English legal rule disallowing hearsay evidence – which corresponded to the growing unwillingness of medical men in their own sphere to rely on published authorities and second-hand facts.

Discussions of medical jurisprudence in the journals of the 1810s and 1820s often made reference to the fact that legal proceedings exposed the uncertainty of medical knowledge. Unlike ordinary practice, where epistemological deficiencies tended to remain hidden, medico legal practice necessarily highlighted such problems. For example, a well-regarded precipitation test for detecting arsenic was shown to be unreliable in the course of the trial of Robert Donnall for murder in 1817, an event which produced consternation in the medical journals.[18] And there were several other trials publicized in the early nineteenth century which illustrated the critical attitude toward evidence that medical improvers wanted to see applied in medicine generally. Reports and discussions of such cases had didactic interest in the context of efforts to reform medical method. The preface to a review of a textbook on medical jurisprudence made this point in 1823:

> The theories of medicine would not have been so proverbially baseless if they had been surveyed with the same minuteness and caution with which medical inquiries at law must be conducted; and we cannot help thinking, that the diffusion of this new branch of knowledge is well calculated to check the growing credulity, the exuberant empiricism, and the habits of hasty induction, which characterize the works of many modern authors in our profession.[19]

Similar observations were made in an article 'On the nature and importance of medical jurisprudence' published in 1820, which pointed out that legal rules of evidence would be 'advantageously applied to medical reasoning in general; and would contribute in no small degree to banish those vague and hypothetical doctrines which have so long retarded the progress of medicine'. By a 'general cultivation and liberal encouragement of this department of medicine', therefore, 'the immediate improvement of the science [of medicine] itself would be promoted'.[20] Forensic medicine could thus be presented as a kind of ideal with respect to the standards of evidence appropriate to the objective, certain, scientific knowledge that reformers envisaged for medicine in general.

The medical journals also presented forensic medicine as a field that was pre-eminently scientific in its subject matter. It dealt with areas of study that were strongly identified with scientific medicine – particularly chemistry and pathological anatomy. In its explanatory goals, too, forensic medicine was notably 'scientific', for it was concerned almost entirely with establishing causation, and not with the task of healing at all. The strength of these associations is evident in a review of 1819 which took exception to physician Gilbert Blane's definition of medicine as 'an ART, – a term, the import of which consists in the adaptation of means to ends'. The reviewer insisted that medicine was also a *science*, and he chose to illustrate the point by means of an example which resembled a typical medico-legal case. He described a hypothetical instance of a man dying with symptoms of brain disorder some days after a blow from a sharp instrument had separated the outer membrane of the skull from the bone, without damaging the parts below, the eventual death being followed by dissection and the discovery of a diseased state of the internal membrane lining the skull. The description of these things, declared the reviewer, constitutes only natural history, and 'cannot properly be termed science (in the received meaning of that term)'. An adequate account of the phenomenon, he went on, requires an 'explanation of the causes of the results': knowledge of the pathway of circulation and a description of the chain of mechanical processes that deprived the skull's internal membrane of its supply of essential fluids. Such an account, which explains why the separation of the outer membrane was necessarily followed by the death of the internal one,

> constitutes science, just as certainly as the explaining why, in a right-angled triangle, the square of its hypotenuse is equal to the square of the two other sides. And, though the object of this knowledge is the application of medicinal agents to the cure of disease, yet the faculty of using those agents with precision cannot be acquired without this kind of knowledge.[21]

Medicine, the reviewer thus urged, required science as well as art, science in the sense of demonstrable knowledge that was not directly related to therapeutic practice but would decisively clarify questions of causation by explicating physiological processes.

Many medical practitioners did not share the reviewer's conviction of the utility of morbid anatomy as a foundation for medical practice. The author of the annual 'Sketch of the progress of medical science' in the preceding volume of the journal pointed out that there was great diversity of opinion on this question.[22] Another reviewer observed in 1828 that although knowledge of morbid anatomy gave 'confidence to the practitioner in the pursuit of his profession', its usefulness in guiding treatment was overrated.[23] Medical jurisprudence, however, was a field of medical practice in which the value and importance of morbid anatomy could not be denied. In fact, a post-mortem investigation for a coroner's inquest represented a direct practical application of the skills and information acquired in the dissecting room.

The science of chemistry, too, was attracting interest and raising expectations among medical men during these years, for the chemical analysis of bodily fluids appeared to offer objective, visible, and measurable facts in the place of qualities that were inferred or subjectively perceived.[24] Those who sought more certainty for medicine were particularly attracted by the potential of chemical science to illuminate the nature and effects of therapeutic substances. Concrete illustrations of the relevance of the new chemistry to medical practice were sparse. Toxicology, however, seemed to be making rapid strides, especially in the detection of mineral poisons, and it had an obvious role to play in the criminal courtroom.

Forensic medicine was thus a field of professional activity in which progress in chemistry and morbid anatomy could have immediate practical relevance; it was one of a very few areas in which the medical sciences could be seen really to matter. The administration of justice might be peripheral to the concerns of medicine, but it was an area in which the power and excitement of scientific medicine could be unambiguously demonstrated. Forensic medicine consequently made an exemplary focus for journal editors seeking to inspire enthusiasm and industry with respect to the medical sciences in general.

As well as being promoted as a demonstrably useful medical science, forensic medicine was presented during this period as a gentlemanly accoutrement for medical practitioners, a desirable accomplishment like a classical education or knowledge of medical history. Mastery of such subjects indicated high social status, for it signified a liberal education and leisure for intellectual pursuits. Forensic medicine in early nineteenth-century Britain consequently had the attractive character of being a new field associated with the very latest in the medical sciences, which nevertheless also had a distinguished learned past in the Continental scholarship on legal medicine dating from the sixteenth century. Displays of erudition in the form of medico-legal history appeared occasionally in the medical journals, providing this branch of medicine with learned connotations, and the absence of indigenous scholarship on forensic medicine was described in 1818 as an 'unseemly void . . . in the medical literature of Britain'.[25]

Noble imagery of the medical jurist affirmed the dignified, gentlemanly character of the field. In his treatise on medical ethics of 1803, Thomas Percival portrayed the performance of medico-legal tasks as a civic obligation which the learned physician should graciously discharge. John Ayrton Paris, distinguished fellow of the College of Physicians who co-authored a textbook on forensic medicine in the 1820s, described his first contribution to the field as a case of *noblesse oblige*. It was a paper about the detection of arsenic which he read to the Royal Geological Society of Cornwall in 1817, the gist of which was reported in the *Medical and Physical Journal*. Paris began by stating that, since a recent notorious poisoning trial in that neighbourhood, his opinion had been so 'repeatedly solicited' on the subject of arsenic tests that he considered it his 'duty' to explore the matter and offer the community his results.[26] Here was no self-promotion, no quackish seeking of publicity, no partisan interest; rather, Paris's introductory vignette was of a man of science being importuned to lend his valuable expertise to a matter of public importance and concern. The task of providing medical testimony in a court of law was given a similar aura of medical condescension and public gratefulness in many idealized representations of the activity that appeared in the medical periodicals.

The portrayal of expertise in forensic medicine as the hallmark of a truly superior practitioner appeared with a different emphasis, which was equally pervasive in the early nineteenth century, in a review of a textbook on medical jurisprudence published in the *Lancet* in 1825. A long preface to the review lamented the rarity of the physician of 'enlarged views, refined judgment and extensive erudition'. The writer then inveighed against the growth of specialisms in surgery as a development degrading to the profession, tending to produce '*artificial* or *partial*, instead of *scientific* or *universal* practitioners'. Surgeons, he urged, should not allow their dominions to be carved up by 'as many petty sovereigns as can find a niche in which to erect their thrones'. After four columns in this vein, the reviewer finally got to the subject of the book under review – forensic medicine – and declared that it 'undoubtedly ought to form a part of every well-conducted medical education'.[27]

Forensic medicine was often promoted in this manner by medical journalists, with explicit reference to it as an example of the expanded education appropriate to a properly scientific profession. The new field could symbolize extensive medical training not only because it was an arcane body of knowledge in itself, but also because it required thorough familiarity with everything a scientific practitioner was supposed to know. When a medical man assisted in judicial proceedings over a case of suspected poisoning, for example, 'the whole of his elementary studies are called into operation, general anatomy, physiology, semeiology, pathology and chemistry'.[28] In the vision of one editor, forensic medicine ranged 'over the vast field of medical erudition, extending through the several regions of the universe, the animal, vegetable, gaseous and mineral kingdoms . . . comprehending the whole of the fascinating sciences included in medicine'.[29] Furthermore, as commentators occasionally noted, when a medical man gave an opinion in a court of law he necessarily drew on the aggregate stock of his professional experience. To be a competent medical jurist, it was necessary to be well-informed in the whole of medical science. Thus glossed, forensic medicine was not just another opportunistic new specialism being hailed by its enthusiasts, but a field which exemplified the educational ideal for the general practitioner.

Another appealing feature of forensic medicine – as the idea was presented in the medical press during these years – was that it assigned a position of public authority and social importance to the medical profession. The medical press frequently remarked on the great value to society of this branch of medicine. Editors and reviewers enlarged on the theme of 'the importance of the application of medical knowledge in aid of the righteous administration of the laws'. Also commonplace was exhilarating prose about how 'the life, the liberties, the rights, and honour of individuals' depended upon protection that the medical profession could provide. Cases in which medical knowledge had overturned the erroneous conclusions of laymen at coroner's inquests were presented as demonstrations of the public utility of 'the right application of professional science'. The objects of forensic medicine were thus 'elevated and important', and, as one reviewer explained, the 'alliance between medicine and justice . . . exalts the dignity of the healing art'.[30] In performing medico-legal duties, practitioners were raised above the self-interested scramble of the medical marketplace and partook of the dignity of the judicial function. They were not advocates, but impartial men of science who contributed learned judgement and experience from a high social position of weighty responsibility. Such functions, in their ideal forms, had tremendous symbolic appeal for those who sought collective gentility and public respect for the medical profession. They displayed clearly, in a public forum, that medicine had a valuable social application worthy of public esteem.

Forensic medicine, then, appealed to journal editors and to other medical improvers for reasons that went beyond its intrinsic importance. It was in several respects a paradigm of scientific medicine and all that that meant. Its subject matter made it an exemplary medical science, for chemistry and morbid anatomy were its principal tools and questions of causation, evidence, and certainty were paramount in medico-legal practice. At the same time, the imposition of legal procedures and standards of proof on forensic medicine made it 'of all the medical sciences . . . the most precise and exact', and therefore an example to be emulated with respect to method.[31] It was a new field of inquiry with a clear research programme, in which significant advances could be made relatively quickly. As for its associated social qualities, not even chemistry in this period could match the capacity of forensic medicine to be both ornamental, gentlemanly, and interesting to amateurs on the one hand, and demonstrably valuable to society in a utilitarian, even Benthamite sense on the other.[32] The role of medical witness was, moreover, often construed as an elevated office of public service. And because of its exceptional visibility in a public forum the practice of forensic medicine had the potential to win for the profession the gratitude and respect of the public at large.

Medico-legal exposures

Thus the ideals. The reality of forensic medicine fell far short of the promise that could be perceived in the new field. For one thing, the actual status of medical expertise in the courts left much to be desired in terms of dignity and authority. Medical witnesses testified on the same footing as other witnesses, and whether medical opinion had any influence on a verdict depended entirely upon the willingness of lay arbiters – the jury, assisted by the judge or the coroner – to be guided by it in that instance. Journal editors often drew attention to cases in which medical judgement had been denied or disregarded. A common source of complaint was the perceived lack of respect for medical testimony in trials for infanticide. The medical test of still-birth was a matter of removing the lungs from the body and placing them in water; floating was thought to indicate that the child had breathed, sinking that it had not. This test, devised on the Continent in the late seventeenth century and applied frequently in British courts thereafter, was widely distrusted among medical practitioners themselves by the late eighteenth century. William Hunter's essay of 1783 'On the uncertainty of the signs of murder, in the case of bastard children' argued that the test was unreliable, and it was explicitly dismissed as inadequate in the 1791 edition of the leading legal textbook on the law of evidence.[33] The test nevertheless continued to be performed, and during the early nineteenth century it regained medical favour. Judges, however, considered the lungs test to have been decisively exploded, and juries tended to be unwilling in any case to convict women of infanticide, for it carried a statutory death penalty. Despite insistence by some medical witnesses (and by the medical press) that the lungs test had been refined and vindicated, and that additional signs of violent death could be reliably detected in newborns, infanticide evidence nevertheless became a subject 'almost of *contention* between courts and professional witnesses, particularly where the latter have shown superior intelligence, and have manifested a desire to perform their duty properly'.[34] A typical observation on the subject was made in 1826 by a reviewer who noted that this part of medico-legal practice was 'never exercised without great hazard of the reputation, and certain laceration of the feelings, even to the most conscientious practitioners'.[35]

During the 1810s and 1820s, the medical periodicals indignantly reported cases in which coroners refused to allow the test, or in which the medical evidence of still-birth was disregarded by judges and juries. In 1824 the editors of the *Medical Repository* described an infanticide inquest in which the coroner's summing-up of the physical question consisted of a mere statement of the opposition between the lay and medical witnesses:

> The coroner, in addressing the jury, is represented to have observed, that they were reduced to a considerably difficulty as to the fact of the child's being born alive or not, it appearing, *from the evidence of the maid-servants* that this was not the case; but if they looked to that of the Surgeon, he would ask whether they were not convinced that the child *was* born alive, and that immediate means were taken to deprive it of life, and prevent respiration?
>
> After a very long discussion, the jury returned a verdict that the child was STILL-BORN!!

The editors elaborated on their use of italics:

> We do not profess to know much about the law of evidence; but . . . we are urged to express some surprise at the evidence of the women being placed in the balance against that of the Surgeon, who seems to have accurately examined into the *best* proofs of vitality under such circumstances. . . . We regret, for the sake of science, as well as justice, that so palpable a case is not likely to undergo a more formal and minute investigation.[36]

Later that year, in their account of a case of suspected infanticide that did reach the trial stage, the editors again expressed their 'regret to say that the judge interfered with regard to the validity of the hydrostatic test, in a manner that baffles our comprehension' and their wish 'that he had not spoken as he did on the pure physiological questions'.[37]

There was similar denial of medical authority in trials for malpractice. In 1824 the *Medical Repository* reported at length a successful lawsuit against a physician for administering excessive amounts of mercury. The editors drew 'the notice of our readers to this trial, because we have seldom met with one in which the interests of the profession have been more decidedly and singularly assailed'. They maintained that the defendant's prescriptions had been within the bounds of prudence, and that the propriety of the treatment could not be doubted by 'any impartial and well-informed Practitioner'. The editors objected to the way the judge had simply passed the mercury question on to the jury without comment, when jurymen were, 'of all the others, least qualified to form any opinion whatever' on whether twenty-two ounces of mercury over nine months was too much.[38]

Lack of deference to medical judgement in the courtroom was not limited to the morally and scientifically problematic areas of infanticide and malpractice. Any inquest was a potential site of lay–medical discord. After a widely-reported poisoning trial in 1818, the *Medical Repository* made a solemn 'protest against that reprehensible and indecorous interference, on the part of the Coroner and Jury, with the business of dissection, which has so justly excited the complaints of Mr. Valentine', the editors themselves having been 'more than once subjected to such interruptions, not less provoking and indecent in themselves, than prejudicial to the interests of justice and science'.[39] Disrespectful treatment of medical witnesses by officials was resented. A correspondent of the *London Medical and Surgical Journal* related two instances known to him in which medical practitioners refused to attend patients thought to have taken poison because they did not want to risk involvement in coroner's inquests. He declared that few medical men would treat cases of this kind, for they were 'unwilling to subject themselves to the insults and petty authority of every Jack-in-office and his satellites, losing their time without the slightest prospects of remuneration'.[40]

Another source of discomfort was professional cross-examination, which could discredit medical testimony by what practitioners considered foul means as well as fair. Several writers observed that medical witnesses were disadvantaged by their passive role under interrogation in an unfamiliar context. A reviewer for the *Edinburgh Medical and Surgical Journal* observed in 1809 that a recent poisoning trial had revealed how medical witnesses could be 'betrayed into apparent contradiction or ignorance in their opinions, by unexpected and artfully contrived questions'.[41] In 1823, a reviewer in the same journal warned practitioners against 'a very common practice (especially with English counsel), of endeavouring to extract opinions on detached points of evidence in succession, and of shunning all inquiry as to the import of the whole collectively', the consequence being that in 'a vast proportion of cases, – for example, in all questions of insanity, infanticide, and poisoning, the witness may be made to express the very opposite of his real opinion'.[42] Writers occasionally complained also of the 'ignorant and unreasonable' pressure exerted on witnesses to reduce their opinions to an unambiguous yes or no.[43] It was pointed out that, whereas a witness was often derided if he equivocated, he appeared untrustworthy if he succumbed to the demand for firm statements and then allowed exceptions to be wrung out of him by cross-examination.[44]

The realities of providing medical expertise in courts of law could thus be a far cry from the pleasing scenes evoked in the advertisements for the new field. Medical journalists of the period complained energetically about the defects they perceived in the legal procedures by which medical evidence was obtained. Even more unsatisfactory in their eyes, however, was the poor quality of much medical testimony itself. Most writers on the subject commented on the general failure of medical practitioners to acquit themselves creditably in court. In 1818 a review in the *Edinburgh Medical and Surgical Journal* pointed out that, although post-mortem dissections were often obstructed by coroners and sheriffs, instances where the discovery of truth was prevented by ignorance on the part of medical witnesses were 'far more numerous':

> We every day hear of medical practitioners giving their evidence with the utmost confidence, on points, which, it is obvious, they never considered with the requisite

> attention; stating facts as universal which admit of many exceptions and modifications; or rejecting them altogether, because exceptions do exist; and destroying evidence, or failing to discover it, from not knowing where it is to be found, nor how it is to be obtained.[45]

Similar observations were made in the *Medical and Physical Journal* by a reviewer who found it 'painful to admit', but undeniable, that 'the records of forensic medicine contain too many examples where medical testimony, instead of clearing doubts, removing obscurities, and furthering the ends of justice, has involved the case in greater perplexity, and tended either to paralyze the arm of the law, or to direct it to an innocent victim'.[46] An account of one such example began: 'A trial took place at Lincoln, on the 12th of last month, characterised by the very common occurrence of medical failure in the article of evidence.'[47] Another summarized an inquest into a case of suspected poisoning reported in the *Morning Chronicle* in 1823, in which erroneous medical testimony appeared to have been influential: 'A Surgeon stated that . . . *had poison been administered*, it would have been observable by the distortion of the face: that, however, was not the case. The jury *expressed themselves satisfied with that opinion*, and returned a verdict of – "Died by the visitation of God." . . . I could mention numerous instances of mischief occasioned by such testimony.'[48]

Great emphasis was placed on the adverse effects of faulty medical testimony on the reputation of the profession as a whole. Indeed, the importance of the study of medical jurisprudence for medicine's public image was a persistent theme in the coverage the field received in the medical journals. Reference was made to 'those disreputable blunders made in our courts', and to the importance of medico-legal knowledge for 'the dignity of the faculty' and 'the character of the Profession generally'.[49] One writer expressed the hope in 1823 that the appearance of the textbook on forensic medicine that he was reviewing would make 'these mortifying exhibitions among the members of our profession less frequent';[50] another perceived in the state of medico-legal practice the 'necessity of doing something compulsory for the redemption of the professional character'.[51] The subject was described in an essay on medical topography as 'a branch of knowledge intimately connected with the respectability of the profession'.[52]

The tendency of medical witnesses to contradict each other was seen as particularly deplorable in this regard. Most medico-legal *causes célèbres* of this period became such because the expert witnesses involved vehemently disagreed. A review in the *Medical Repository* for 1821 observed that medical opinion in courts of law had acquired 'the stigma of being more discrepant and discordant than any other', and declared that it was 'expedient' for the profession 'to do all in our power to diminish the justness of the accusation'.[53] A trial report entitled 'Charge of rape. Discrepancy of medical evidence, with remarks', published in 1830, observed that during the preceding year 'the conflicting testimony of medical men in this city, has been quite sufficient to bring the character of the profession to the lowest degree of humiliation, if not contempt'.[54] A letter about a poisoning trial in 1825 expressed 'regret that medical men should ever be opposed to one another in their evidence given in courts of justice'. A difference of opinion in such circumstances, the writer explained, tended 'to expose the most useful and honourable of all professions to the sneers of prejudice and ignorance', and had the effect of 'lessening medical science in the esteem and confidence of the public'.[55]

This emphasis on the importance of medico-legal practice for the reputation of the profession was not 'empty' rhetoric. It was replete with significance in a period in which the medical profession appears to have been preoccupied with its image. Concern was often expressed in the medical periodicals of the early nineteenth century about the standing of medicine in the estimation of the public. According to one journal editor, writing in 1830, 'public confidence in the healing art' had been 'so much injured of late, that many deprive themselves of its aid altogether'. A year later a review in the same journal observed that 'the medical profession will be long ere it is raised to that rank in society which it merits', for 'complaints are continually made of the manner in which we are regarded, and of the rapid progress *downwards*, which we are making in the eyes of the unprofessional public'.[56] A pervasive analysis of this alleged decline of medical authority and status focused on the educational attainments of the bulk of practitioners and found the profession wanting. During the 1810s and 1820s, complaints about the ignorance of duly qualified medical men were almost as common in the medical press as were expressions of indignation about the pretensions of irregulars.

The causes of these problems were thought to lie in the 'glaring defects' of 'the Medical Government in this country', especially as these affected education.[57] The medical corporations responsible for licensing most regular practitioners were slow to bring their training requirements in line with the scientific ideals of reformers. The obligation of apothecaries and surgeons to serve an apprenticeship was objected to as embodying a pre-scientific, craft-orientated method of professional training which prevented the extension of the period of formal education in lecture halls and hospitals. Training in an important part of general practice – midwifery – was not required by any corporation until 1827, an omission which, the medical press repeatedly pointed out, resulted in grossly incompetent midwifery practice. During the 1820s there was criticism of the alleged superficiality of the qualifying examinations conducted by the College of Surgeons and the Society of Apothecaries. The nepotism by which hospital posts were distributed was bitterly resented, as was the anachronistic snobbery that denied general practitioners full membership of the College of Surgeons and College of Physicians. Rules enacted by the College of Surgeons in 1822 and 1824, which discriminated against private medical schools and increased the hospital élite's control of teaching, were denounced as acts of corruption which had compromised the quality of education in anatomy and surgery. Training in dissection was expensive, for most of the bodies had to be obtained illegally, and legislation to ensure a supply for medical teaching was not forthcoming until 1832. These obstacles to the formation of a well-educated, meritocratic profession were repeatedly complained of in the medical periodicals, and form the backdrop against which journalistic commentary on forensic medicine needs to be viewed.[58]

A common feature of the various perspectives on medical improvement was concern about the social status of the profession. In its summary of the aims of the long series of meetings and parliamentary bills that preceded the Apothecaries' Act of 1815, the *Medical and Physical Journal* emphasized rank and dignity as much as the exclusion of the unqualified. The activists were seeking, it explained,

> to meliorate the science of medicine, to improve the condition of those properly employed in it, to suppress cheats and imposters, to protect honest merit, and to reward

> talent. To see the healing art rescued from the mean and degrading circumstances in which it was often found . . . to place it in a station which its importance demanded, and to protect it by wholesome and rational laws which its usefulness deserved.[59]

Efforts were made through the medical press during these years to raise standards of conduct among regular practitioners in the interests of collective reputation. Editorials, articles, and letters voiced disapproval of practices considered degrading to an honourable profession, such as the advertisement of cures, incivility towards fellow practitioners, even an uneducated or vulgarly exuberant style in professional writing.[60] The interdependency of members of the profession with respect to reputation was often stressed. Easy entrance to the regular profession was claimed to be swelling its ranks with ill-educated practitioners, with the result that conscientious, scientific practitioners became associated with a large mass of unworthy yet formally qualified ones. In 1824 a surgeon-apothecary wrote to the editors of the *Medical Repository* as the 'censors of medical conduct', complaining of the traffic in patent medicines by regular surgeons and apothecaries. Legislation, he said, could protect against the intrusions of uneducated pretenders, but what of those 'of our order who have lost sight of what they owe to themselves, to their brethren, and to society'? The correspondent declared that as a member of the profession he was personally injured by practitioners who thus debased it, and he urged the profession 'to rouse itself to the assertion of its dignity'. The editors responded by pointing to steps they had been taking to foster the respectability of the professional character.[61]

In the context of these concerns about professional image and collective dignity, the performance of medical witnesses in trial proceedings was important. Such proceedings were public in a way that ordinary medical practice was not, giving forensic medicine unique visibility. The accounts of medical testimony at inquests and trials that appeared in newspapers were consequently viewed by medical journalists as highly relevant to the profession's public relations. Exposures of ignorance and error on the part of some practitioners were perceived as an embarrassment to all. Many trial reports, reviews, and articles on forensic medicine in the medical press alluded to its significance in this respect. A correspondent of the *Lancet* lamented in 1826, 'It is seldom . . . we read medical evidence that is worthy of the members of a yclept liberal profession'; he proceeded to describe the inadequate medical evidence given at two recent trials, in the hope, he said, 'of exciting the attention of the profession for their own *credit* to medical jurisprudence'.[62] The *Medical Repository* reported an inquest on the body of a man struck by lightning in 1824 by printing a long passage from a non-medical periodical which had criticized the casual and unscientific nature of the post-mortem. The *Repository*'s editors considered it a matter to which 'the attention of the Profession should be drawn. . . . Our brethren will see that the eyes of all men are upon them, as to the manner in which they discharge their medico-legal duties.' Although the editors acknowledged that the legal purposes of the particular inquest had been perfectly well served by the superficial post-mortem and the imprecise medical testimony, 'we still would say that, as it was judged necessary to call on a medical practitioner for his opinion as to the cause of death, the practitioner should have taken all due pains to have formed one, and not have spoken so vaguely'.[63] From the perspective of the *Medical Repository*, the legal function of forensic medicine was not its only significance; the issues themselves mattered as questions of science, and so did the quality of medical testimony liable to be placed in public view. Similar concerns were expressed in the *London Medical and Surgical Journal*'s report of a malpractice trial in 1830:

> We should strongly advise some of the medical men who figured in this inquiry, to look into some work on medical jurisprudence, before their next appearance in a court of justice, and also to peruse some standard work on the question on which they intend to give evidence. One would think science had fled from the profession, when its members come before their contemporaries and the public, and broach the most heterodox and absurd opinions.[64]

The common ground between a concern with professional reform and the promotion of this field of study is well illustrated by the editors' preface to some excerpts from a textbook on forensic medicine that were printed in the *Medical Repository* in 1825. Several of the reformist themes discussed above –

insufficient education, declining social status, the culpable inaction of the medical corporations, the link between science and respectability, unworthy conduct among the profession's lower ranks – were interwoven in a single passage arguing for compulsory training in forensic medicine:

> [T]he great importance which the . . . literary tribunals of the country have attached . . . to this particular application of medical science, proves the propriety of requiring from the professional student a regular course of study of it. It is to be hoped that, at a period when the numbers of those entering upon the prosecution of medical studies are so very great . . . the constituted guardians of the Profession will exert the very efficient means they have in their power, of at least preventing its respectability from degenerating. . . . [T]hey should require respectively that those entering upon professional studies . . . shall previously have obtained a much more liberal education than is at present thought necessary by many. . . . If this important matter be not better attended to . . . our science will degenerate into a cunning craft. . . .

The preface concluded by urging the medical corporations that in addition to 'a sufficient number of full courses of instruction in every department of medical knowledge, attendance be also required on lectures on medical jurisprudence', the importance of the latter being 'now so apparent as not to admit of dispute'.[65]

Publicity, reform, and forensic medicine

The medical press exaggerated the pitfalls awaiting an uninformed medical witness, of course, in its efforts to demonstrate the 'imperious necessity' of training in legal medicine.[66] Criminal trial records of the early nineteenth century do not reveal the degree of frustration and failure said by medico-legal publicists to occur 'every day' and at 'every assize'.[67] However, wide publicity was given to trial proceedings through newspapers and magazines, and any medical testimony was well covered. The *Lancet* observed drily in 1832 that the reward for conducting a post-mortem for a coroner's inquest was 'the glory of creating a paragraph in the morning papers'.[68]

The medical press itself played a deliberately active role in publicizing the cases of medico-legal difficulty that did occur. In 1819 the *Medical Repository* described the imperfect application and appreciation of 'the science of juridical medicine' as an 'evil' in the 'present system of legislation' which deserved the attention of reformers; for its part, the *Repository* considered that 'to expose the malignity of its operation' would 'serve as the first step towards arresting its progress'.[69] Several years later, in announcing their intention to report trials and inquests involving medical testimony more assiduously, the editors declared that they would not be concealing displays of 'ignorance and disregard of the dignity and true interests of the Profession' because they conceived it their duty 'to hold up the culpable individual as a warning to the whole community'.[70] Editors emphasized the absence of malice in this policy, reminding one victim that 'his evidence, and that of all the other medical men, are fair subjects for impartial criticism', and asking him to bear in mind that 'our talented contemporary, the Med. Chir. Rev. and the Med. Gazette, have been much more caustic on the occasion than ourselves'.[71] They had 'no object in view, but the promotion of the dignity of our profession and the interests of humanity'.[72]

This strategy of reforming by exposing defects was commonly employed in the medical journals. Most notoriously, the *Lancet* editor Thomas Wakley sought out and publicized cases of incompetent hospital practice in order to denounce corruption and force change.[73] The *London Medical and Surgical Journal* practised a less aggressive but equally persistent 'system of remonstrance, by which we hope to expedite the approach of the day when the Profession . . . shall be placed on a better footing', and its editor considered the exposure of inadequacy to be an effective tool of medical reform.[74] Reviewing a chemical work on pharmacology in 1831, the journal observed that the London College of Physicians had always been 'in the rear of the march of science', and declared that if the rest of the medical press 'had only spirit to speak the truth, and that openly, the medical rulers in England would cease to be behind all their contemporaries in other nations'.[75]

The question of the significance of medico-legal exposures was discussed by Wakley in his preamble to an inquest report in

1832. It had been recently observed, he said, that the sure test of 'the state of professional knowledge' in any nation was 'the character of the medical testimony in its forensic investigations'. Wakley saw 'much truth in this opinion – mortifying as the sequel may show its application to the state of British medicine to be'. However, he pointed out that the legal system itself was partly to blame for the crowding of coroner's courts with 'incompetent, juvenile, babbling, medical witnesses' because there was no legal rule to ensure that medico-legal investigations were conducted by practitioners with competence in forensic medicine.[76] Wakely repeatedly urged that coroners should be medically qualified, and he campaigned vigorously for legislation to provide for the payment of medical witnesses. The *Lancet*'s medico-legal content was consequently often orientated towards reforming the medico-legal system itself, and similar purposes can be discerned in other journals under titles like 'Rupture of the liver – ignorance of lawyer coroners'.[77] The concern of this chapter, however, has been to show how the subject of forensic medicine could function as a rhetorical resource of much wider application.

It seems clear that the zeal with which forensic medicine was promoted in medical periodicals during these years was inspired partly by its associations with the cause of medical improvement and reform. A combination of features peculiar to forensic medicine made it an apt emblem of the goals of the self-consciously progressive medical men who edited and contributed to professional journals. With regard to both subject matter and epistemology, forensic medicine was a model and an example of scientific medicine. At the same time, medico-legal practice was one of the very few instances in which medical expertise was called upon independently of the practice of healing, and in which professional knowledge was considered in isolation from the issue of therapeutic effectiveness. The new field could therefore demonstrate the power of the medical sciences, and it could do so in a highly public manner. As an idea, forensic medicine also implied and symbolized an attractive professional character: it was arcane, but also necessary; gentlemanly, but utilitarian. Properly regulated, the practice of forensic medicine offered to the profession a highly acceptable role of public importance and authority.

If the idea of forensic medicine exemplified some of the goals of medical improvers, contemporary medico-legal practice illustrated many of the defects that preoccupied reformers: the ineffective regulation of medical practice, the inadequate training of practitioners in dissection and pathological anatomy, the rivalry and dogmatism for which medicine was notorious, and the sheer uncertainty of a science that could generate disagreement and ambiguity so persistently. The practice of forensic medicine was also thought to demonstrate, with exceptional concreteness and clarity, how the precarious reputation of the profession as a whole could be affected by the conduct and ability of individual members. Most medico-legal cases were thus, one way or another, grist for the reformist mill, and their value in this respect brought them notice in the medical press. The fact that forensic medicine could illustrate and exemplify both the ideals and the grievances of medical reformers during the early nineteenth century made it an attractive subject for medical writers who were dedicated to improving their profession.

Notes

1. Society of Apothecaries MS. 8239, 'Court of Examiners, Minutes', vol. IV (1828–33), 27 August 1829, 9 September 1830, Guildhall Library.

2. George Clark, *A History of the Royal College of Physicians*, 2 vols (Oxford, 1966), vol. II, p. 649; *A Statement by the Society of Apothecaries, on the Subject of their Administration of the Apothecaries Act* (1844), p. 16; S. W. F. Holloway, 'The Apothecaries' Act, 1815: a reinterpretation', *Medical History*, 10 (1966), 107–29, 221–36, p. 235.

3. Michael Ryan, 'Observations on the importance of medical jurisprudence', *London Medical and Surgical Journal*, 4 (1830), 41–7, p. 43. Ryan was referring to the recommendation of August 1829; the enactment of September 1830 had not yet occurred.

4. W. Royston, 'Hints for a medical topography of Great Britain', *London Medical and Physical Journal*, 21 (1809), 1–16, 91–102, pp. 99–100.

5. 'Address to the Faculty', *London Medical Repository*, 1 (1814), 1–16, pp. 5–6.

6. Books on forensic medicine also mushroomed in Britain during this sixteen-year period; Thomas Forbes gives a chronological list which includes most of them in *Surgeons at the Bailey: English Forensic Medicine to 1878* (New Haven, 1985), pp. 231–2. The extensive periodical literature on the subject published during these years has not been commented on by historians.

7. *London Medical Repository*, 9 (1818), 128–9, p. 128; 'Medical jurisprudence', *London Medical Repository*, 10 (1818), 508–13, p. 513.

8. 'Address to the Faculty, *London Medical Repository*, n.s., 1 (1824), [xi]–[xiv], p. [xiii]; 'Political medicine: introductory remarks', ibid., 85–90, p. 86.

9. The others I have surveyed are the *London Medical and Physical Journal* (established 1799), the *Edinburgh Medical and Surgical Journal* (established 1805), the *Lancet* (established 1823), and the *London Medical and Surgical Journal* (established 1828).

10. Robert Christison, *The Life of Sir Robert Christison, Bart.*, ed. by his sons (Edinburgh, 1885), vol. I (Autobiography), pp. 337–8.

11. On this theme, see Susan Lawrence, 'Science and medicine at the London hospitals: the development of teaching and research, 1750–1815; PhD thesis, University of Toronto, 1985, pp. 506–7, 558–9.

12. 'Historical sketch of the progress of medicine, from July to December, 1811', *London Medical and Physical Journal*, 27, 2–41, p. 2.

13. *Elements of Medical Logick* (London, 1819), p. 12.

14. William Hutchinson, Review of *General Indications which relate to the laws of the Organic Life*, in 'Historical sketch of the progress of medicine', *London Medical and Physical Journal*, 43 (1820), [i]–xcvi, pp. x, xii.

15. See, for example, 'The time for gathering digitalis', *London Medical and Surgical Journal*, 1 (1828), 199–200; John Gordon Smith, 'Observations on new remedies, and on the oil of croton', *London Medical Repository*, 17 (1822), 8–12, pp. 10–11.

16. *London Medical Gazette*, 7 (1830–1), 363–5.

17. 'Review of *Official Papers relating to Operations performed by Order of the Directors of the Royal Hospital for Seamen at Greenwich . . . for the purpose of ascertaining the general efficacy of the new modes of Treatment practised by Mr. Adams, for the Cure of the Various Species of Cataract, and the Egyptian Ophthalmia*', *Edinburgh Medical and Surgical Journal*, 10 (1814), 395. Emphasis in original.

18. J. Kerr, 'On poisoning with arsenic', *London Medical and Physical Journal*, 38 (1817), 92–5; J. Hume, 'On poisoning with arsenic', ibid., 39 (1818), 27–33; John Prideaux, 'On the tests for arsenic, in reply to Mr. Hume', ibid., 40 (1818), 185–8; 'Test of arsenic', *London Medical Repository*, 8 (1817), 177–8.

19. Review of *Medical Jurisprudence* by J. A. Paris and J. S. M. Fonblanque, *Edinburgh Medical and Surgical Journal*, 19 (1823), 601–30, p. 604.

20. W.M.I., 'Observations on the nature and importance of medical jurisprudence', *London Magazine*, 1 (1820), 132–6, p. 135. Christopher Hamlin has made this point in his discussion of later debates about medical testimony; see his 'Scientific method and expert witnessing: Victorian perspectives on a modern problem', *Social Studies of Science* 16 (1986), 485–513.

21. Review of *Elements of Medical Logick* by Gilbert Blane, *London Medical and Physical Journal*, 42 (1819), 301–14, 390–9, p. 304.

22. 'Historical sketch of the progress of medical science, from June 1818, to January 1819', *London Medical and Physical Journal*, 41 (1819), 1–72, p. 9.

23. Review of *An Essay on a New Mode of Treatment for Diseased Joints*

by Thomas Buchanan, *London Medical and Surgical Journal*, 1 (1828), 503–18, pp. 503–4.

24. Susan Lawrence, 'Science and medicine at the London hospitals', pp. 560–3, 606–9.

25. For example, the lengthy 'review' of the second edition of *Elements of Juridical or Forensic Medicine* by George Edward Male in the *London Medical Repository*, 12 (1819), 415–31, is almost entirely compossed of a historical overview of forensic medicine. Quotation: 'Medical Jurisprudence', *London Medical Repository*, 10 (1818), 508–13, p. 513.

26. 'Royal Geological Society of Cornwall', *London Medical and Physical Journal*, 38 (1817), 172–3.

27. Review of *Elements of Medical Jurisprudence* by T.R. Beck, *Lancet* 6 (1825), 172–80, pp. 172–4. Emphasis in original.

28. Review of *A Treatise on Poisons* by Robert Christison and *An Essay on the Operation of Poisonous Agents upon the Living Body* by John Morgan, *London Medical Surgical Journal*, 4 (1830), 265–84, p. 269, paraphrasing Christison.

29. Michael Ryan, 'Of the utility and importance of the study of state medicine', *London Medical and Surgical Journal*, 4 (1830), 217–24, p. 219.

30. The phrases quoted in this paragraph are from the following: Review of *The Principles of Forensic Medicine* by J. G. Smith, *London Medical and Physical Journal*, 52 (1824), 135–48, 223–40, p. 135; Smith, 'Forensic medicine: case of the late Mr. Neale and Butler, the soldier, medico-legally considered', *Lancet* 2 (1828–9), 84–8; Smith, *The Claims of Forensic Medicine* (London, 1829), p. 14; Review of *Elements of Juridical or Forensic Medicine* (2nd edn) by G. E. Male, *London Medical Repository*, 12 (1819), 415–31, p. 416.

31. Review of *Medical Jurisprudence* by J. A. Paris and J. S. M. Fonblanque, *Edinburgh Medical and Surgical Journal*, 19 (1823), 601–30, p. 604.

32. Morris Berman has argued for the contemporary currency of a utilitarian ideology of science, especially chemistry, in *Social Change and Scientific Organization: The Royal Institution, 1799–1844* (Ithaca, NY, 1978), ch. 4.

33. *Medical Observations and Inquiries*, 6 (1783), 266–90; Capel Lofft (ed.), *The Law of Evidence, by Lord Chief Baron Gilbert*, 4 vols (London, 1791), vol. I, p. 301.

34. John Gordon Smith, *Hints for the Examination of Medical Witnesses* (London, 1829), p. 70. Emphasis in original.

35. 'Marks of vitality in new-born infants', *London Medical and Physical Journal*, 55 (1826), 527–8, p. 528.

36. 'Infanticide', *London Medical Repository*, n.s., 1 (1824), 344–7, pp. 345–6. Emphasis in original.

37. 'Infanticide', *London Medical Repository*, n.s., 2 (1824), 258.

38. 'Case of Leach *v.* Veitch', *London Medical Repository*, n.s., 1 (1824), 172–7.

39. 'Medical jurisprudence', *London Medical Repository*, 10 (1818),

508–13, p. 509.

40. 'Case of poisoning by the Lancaster or black drop, a preparation of opium', *London Medical and Surgical Journal*, 5 (1830), 128–9, p. 128.

41. Review of *The Trial of Charles Angus: A Vindication of the Opinions delivered in Evidence by the Medical Witnesses for the Crown*, and *Remarks on a late Publication, entitled, 'A Vindication of the Opinions, &c'* by James Carson, *Edinburgh Medical and Surgical Journal*, 5 (1809), 220–9, p. 225.

42. Review of *Medical Jurisprudence* by J. A. Paris and J. S. M. Fonblanque, *Edinburgh Medical and Surgical Journal*, 19 (1823), 601–30, p. 611.

43. G. N. Hill, 'Mr. Hill, on the Liverpool controversy', *London Medical and Physical Journal*, 21 (1809), 399–405, pp. 403, 404.

44. 'Case of Leach *v.* Veitch', *London Medical Repository*, n.s., 1 (1824), 172–7, p. 176; 'Extracts from "An Analysis of Medical Evidence, &c."', *London Medical and Physical Journal*, 53 (1825), 213–21, p. 217.

45. Review of *A Treatise on Forensic Medicine* by O. W. Bartley and *An Epitome of Juridical or Forensic Medicine* by G. E. Male, *Edinburgh Medical and Surgical Journal*, 14 (1818), 111–12, p. 111.

46. Review of *The Principles of Forensic Medicine* by J. G. Smith, *London Medical and Physical Journal*, 52 (1824), 135–48, 223–40, p. 136.

47. 'Poisoning by arsenic', *London Medical Repository*, n.s., 1 (1824), 348–9, p. 348.

48. G. E. Male, 'Remarks on the medical evidence adduced on the trial of Captain Donellan, in defence of the author's opinion respecting it', *London Medical Repository*, n.s., 2 (1824), 376–80, p. 379. Emphasis in original.

49. Michael Ryan, 'Of the utility and importance of the study of state medicine', *London Medical and Surgical Journal*, 4 (1830), 217–24, p. 219; Ryan, 'Laws relating to the medical profession', *London Medical and Surgical Journal*, 5 (1830), 313–35, p. 329; Review of *An Analysis of Medical Evidence* by J. G. Smith, *London Medical Repository*, n.s., 3 (1825), 207–27, p. 208.

50. Review of *The Principles of Forensic Medicine* by J. G. Smith, *London Medical and Physical Journal*, 52 (1824), 135–48, 223–40, p. 136.

51. John Gordon Smith, 'Introductory lecture', *London Medical and Surgical Journal*, n.s., 1 (1832), 68–72, p. 71, recalling the period before the Apothecaries' regulation of 1830.

52. W. Royston, 'Hints for a medical topography of Great Britain', *London Medical and Physical Journal*, 21 (1809), 1–16, 91–102, pp. 99–100.

53. Review of *The Principles of Forensic Medicine* by J. G. Smith, *London Medical Repository*, 16 (1821), 211–34, p. 228.

54. *London Medical and Surgical Journal*, 4 (1830), 48–59, p. 48.

55. James Torrie, 'Account of an individual who swallowed a drachm of powdered cantharides', *London Medical and Physical Journal*, 54 (1825), 463–5, p. 465.

56. 'Dr. Ryan on state of the medical profession', *London Medical and Surgical Journal*, 5 (1830), 223–42, p. 224; Review of 'On old

dislocations; being an essay read before the Glasgow Medical Society, 1st Feb. 1831. By James Laurie', *London Medical and Surgical Journal*, 6(1831), 513–18, p. 517.

57. Review of *Suggestions for the Relief of the Sick Poor, and the Improvement of the Medical Profession in Great Britain* by John Dunn, *London Medical Repository*, 9 (1818), 234–6, p. 236.

58. For these themes, see, for example, 'On medical apprenticeships' and 'On the medical profession', *London Medical Repository*, 15 (1821), 89–101 and 353–60; 'Medical and physical intelligence. Royal College of Surgeons in London', *London Medical and Physical Journal*, 51 (1824), 521–4; Adrian Desmond, *The Politics of Evolution: Morphology, Medicine, and Reform in Radical London* (Chicago, 1989), ch. 3; Irvine Loudon, *Medical Care and the General Practitioner 1750–1850* (Oxford, 1986), ch. 4; Ivan Waddington, *The Medical Profession in the Industrial Revolution* (Dublin, 1984), ch. 4.

59. 'Historical sketch of the progress of medicine for the year 1810, and from January to June 1811', *London Medical and Physical Journal*, 26 (1811), 1–38, p. 2–3.

60. Review of *Remarks on Arsenic* by John Marshall, *London Medical Repository*, 8 (1817), 149–63, p. 163; Review of *Medical Ethics* by Thomas Percival, *London Medical and Physical Journal*, 11 (1804), 181–4.

61. 'Medical Police – Professional delinquency', *London Medical Repository*, n.s., 2 (1824), 166–72.

62. Atticus, 'Medical jurisprudence. the Editor of the Lancet', *Lancet*, 11 (1826–27), 393. Emphasis in original.

63. 'Aerostation. – Death of Mr. Harris', *London Medical Repository*, n.s., 2 (1824), 82–3.

64. 'Medical jurisprudence. 11. Shocking effect of quackery in London', *London Medical and Surgical Journal*, 5 (1830), 259–64, p. 263.

65. Review of *An Analysis of Medical Evidence* by J. G. Smith, *London Medical Repository*, n.s., 3 (1825), 207–27, pp. 207–8. Emphasis in original.

66. Michael Ryan, 'Charge of rape. Discrepancy of medical evidence, with remarks', *London Medical and Surgical Journal*, 4 (1830), 48–59, p. 48.

67. Review of *A Treatise on Forensic Medicine* by O. W. Bartley and *An Epitome of Juridical or Forensic Medicine* by (2nd edn) G.E. Male, *Edinburgh Medical and Surgical Journal*, 14 (1818), 111–12, p. 111; John Elliotson, *The Introductory Lecture of a Course upon State-Medicine* (London, 1821), p. 15.

68. 'Forensic medicine as a test of knowledge, *Lancet*, 2 (1831–2), 621–5, p. 621.

69. Review of *Elements of Juridical or Forensic Medicine* (2nd edn), by G. E. Male, *London Medical Repository*, 12 (1819), 415–31, p. 416.

70. 'Political medicine. Introductory remarks', *London Medical Repository*, n.s., 1 (1824), 85–7, p. 87.

71. 'Medical jurisprudence', *London Medical and Surgical Journal*, 5 (1830), 342–52, p. 344.

72. 'Inquest on the body of Miss Cashin', *London Medical and Surgical Journal*, 5 (1830), 406–11, p. 409.

73. S. Squire Sprigge, *The Life and Times of Thomas Wakley* (London, 1897); Mary Bostetter, 'The Journalism of Thomas Wakley', in Joel H. Wiener (ed.), *Innovators and Preachers: The Role of the Editor in Victorian England* (Westport, Connecticut, 1985), pp. 275–92.

74. Untitled editorial, *London Medical and Surgical Journal*, n.s., 1 (1832), 17–18, p. 17.

75. Review of *Observations Chemical and Practical, on the Dublin Pharmacopoeia* by F. Barker and W. F. Montgomery, *London Medical and Surgical Journal*, 6 (1831), 86–110, p. 87.

76. 'Forensic medicine as a test of knowledge', *Lancet* 2 (1831–2), 621–5, p. 621.

77. Dr. Tuthill, 'Rupture of the liver – ignorance of lawyer coroners', *London Medical and Surgical Journal*, 6 (1831), 304–7.

10

Religion, respectability and the origins of the modern nurse

Perry Williams

Our folk history of nursing is dominated by two characters. The first is Sarah Gamp, the comic working-class nurse of Charles Dickens's *Martin Chuzzlewit*: old, fat, gin-swilling, clumsy, always thinking of her own welfare rather than that of her patients. The second character is Florence Nightingale, the 'lady with the lamp' who brought comfort to the wounded soldiers at Scutari Hospital during the Crimean War, who recognized the appalling state of nursing and by her efforts and example created the modern, efficient, dedicated nurse of today. In the popular culture of our society, the story of the origins of the modern nurse is the story of these two characters.[1] Most grand-sweep histories of nursing are still organized around this traditional story, although their telling of it may be more subtle. They are likely, for instance, to introduce further characters, pointing out that Florence Nightingale was not the first to recognize the need for nursing reform; they may mention Elizabeth Fry and her Institute of Nursing Sisters, the St John's House Institution for Nurses, and the French Sisters of Charity and the Béguines communities of Flanders which provided an inspiration and a model for early nursing reformers. The story remains, however, one of progress: from the gross and incompetent nurse of the Sarah Gamp type to the trained and committed nurse personified by Florence Nightingale.[2]

For many of those working in the field of nursing history, this story is something to be rejected and abandoned. The dramatic expansion of the field since 1980, involving many nurses and others with an interest in contemporary health care, was based on the realization that there were things of interest outside the scope of the traditional story: in the more recent past rather than the early nineteenth century, in the experience of ordinary nurses rather than that of great women and men, and in the nursing of the provinces rather than that of London.[3] These new lines of research were valuable, and greatly extended our knowledge of such important matters as the actualities of nurse training and practice and the place of nursing in twentieth-century state health-care provision.[4] As a result, however, the traditional story was abandoned so thoroughly that no effort was devoted to producing a more critical account of the nursing reforms of the first few decades of the nineteenth century. Such critical revision as was done mostly concentrated on Florence Nightingale, and mainly served to show that she was not as important as the traditional story had made out.[5] An account of what *was* important in the origin of the modern nurse – which does seem to lie in this period – is only now being developed.[6] This chapter is meant as a contribution towards such an account, in an attempt to find a more sophisticated and truer story to replace the folk history with which we all grew up.

The problem with the traditional story, most critics would feel, has to do with it being a story of triumphal progress: in effect a Whig history – or more precisely a 'present-centred' – history of nursing.[7] As Celia Davies observes, it is essentially evaluative;[8] indeed, it is fundamentally a moral story, the purpose of whose telling is to communicate certain values rather than provide a causal account of past events. The values therefore appear as eternally true and unproblematic; progress is presented as a simple matter of enlightenment, in a way which makes no sense as a causal account. Consider: according to the story, nurses were very much of the Sarah Gamp type – ignorant, drunk, and lazy – until certain wise and good people introduced nurse training, perhaps on a Continental model. But if nurses were as obviously incompetent as Dickens made Sarah Gamp out to be, then why did nobody do anything about it before the early nineteenth century? The Sisters of Charity and the Béguines had existed for over a hundred years, so why, for most of the eighteenth century, did nobody think of imitating them in England?

The answer must be that no nursing problem was seen. Sarah Gamp was obviously a problematic nurse, but she was a fictional character, the 'old nurse' seen from Dickens's reformer perspective. Nurses were seen differently during the eighteenth century. They were not conceived of as medical practitioners but more as domestic servants; indeed, that was where they were placed in the occupational tables of the national census right up to 1861. Domestic nurses, by far the biggest class, were employed by a household in exactly the same way as servants, for the essentially similar duty of watching over the sick. Even hospital nurses (who made up less than 3 per cent of census-recorded nurses)[9] had duties and an organization similar to that of domestic servants. Their duties as far as patient care was concerned were the manual tasks of administering food and medicine, changing linen and emptying bedpans, and they also did the basic hospital cleaning, including scrubbing the floors. The whole domestic organization was under the direction of a Matron, effectively a housekeeper, recruited from a higher order of society and paid accordingly. The wages of regular nurses varied considerably between different hospitals, most having a differential rate for the senior nurses or sisters[10] in charge of each ward and the watch-women on night duty, but over the period 1780–1830 they were typically in the range of five to ten pounds per annum[11] – comparable with the wages of a domestic servant, and in certain areas lower, with the result that the women who became nurses tended to be those who were unable to get a position in a household. The position of nurses was therefore comparable to that of cleaners today; they were recruited from the lowest rungs of society without any special knowledge or commitment to the job, but since their work was essentially unskilled manual labour there was no necessary reason why employers, whether in households or in hospitals, should have considered this a problem.

The question must be reversed; we should not be asking, why did nobody do anything about nurses for so long?, but rather, why did anybody think it necessary to do something about it in the first place? It is to answer this question that I am returning to the material of the traditional story, the nursing reformers up to and including Florence Nightingale, seeing them now not as the first to be enlightened but as the first to think change necessary, candidates therefore not for celebration but for explanation. Having rejected such vague and question-begging descriptions of their activity as 'progress' or 'reform', the aim will be to find out *what* precisely they were doing and *why*. I will be confining my attention to the nursing reformers who appear in the traditional histories; no doubt there were many other reform schemes which never saw the light of day or left no relics beyond locally circulated pamphlets, but I have found that a survey even of just those events which reached the traditional histories enables some important conclusions to be drawn.

This re-examination of nursing reformers can begin with the hospitals, since many of the official hospital histories include items from their records which seem to be early signs of a newly perceived need for nursing reform. The raising of nurses' wages, for example, was not always just a cost-of-living increase. At the Manchester Royal Infirmary in 1785, the rise was coupled with an order that the nurses should cease their practice of demanding a payment of threepence from each patient on their admission to the hospital and further money thereafter. Understandably, given their low income, nurses at many institutions commonly took bribes from their patients, with the threat of refusing to attend to them. The Royal Infirmary governors, however, now saw this as unacceptable, and were trying to stamp it out.[12] Again, at the Middlesex Hospital in 1838, the raising of nurses' wages had a very explicit purpose, for the governors expressed the hope 'of procuring and retaining the better description of nurses – women who will take more interest in their duties, their character and their appearance'.[13] In other words, the level of commitment, character, and appearance of their nurses was no longer acceptable to the governors, and they saw a solution to this problem in recruiting women from higher up the social scale.

Hospital records for the early nineteenth century also reveal efforts to introduce greater selectivity in the appointment of nurses, typically by requiring all appointments to be approved at a higher administrative level. At Manchester in the 1840s, for example, when a new post of Resident Medical Officer was created, its duties including shared responsibility with the Matron for all nursing appointments and dismissals.[14] Some hospitals attempted to lay down minimum standards for their nurses, but they were often disappointed in their efforts; the London Hospital, for instance, resolved in 1822 to appoint only nurses who could read and write, but it proved impossible to adhere to this strictly.[15]

A number of hospitals instituted administrative changes designed to increase control and discipline over nurses inside the institution. At St. Thomas's Hospital in the early nineteenth century, the Matron, Sarah Savery, began recruiting ward sisters separately instead of promoting ordinary nurses to that rank, thus opening a way for the establishment of new standards among the nurses through the sisters' personal influence and ward discipline.[16] Other matrons, most famously Sarah Wardroper who succeeded Sarah Savery at St. Thomas's, instituted regular clampdowns on drinking among the nurses.[17] Some hospitals, such as Guy's, considered boarding their nurses within the hospital – not for convenience of patient care, but to cope with what the Guy's Superintendent called 'irregularity', which here meant food pilfering.[18] Like taking bribes from patients, this seems to have been common among hospital nurses.

From the steps which hospital governors were taking by the early nineteenth century, we can not only infer that they were increasingly finding their nurses unsatisfactory but also specify the kind of problem that they were now perceiving. Their anxiety was not on the whole about the technical competence of nurses in the manual work of patient care but about their moral standards: their taking money from patients, stealing, drinking, being dirty and untidy, and being generally 'of poor character'. This was a concern entirely characteristic of this period, in which the attitudes of the middling classes were increasingly dominated by evangelicalism.[19] The first signs of concern about nurses' morals appear in the 1780s and 1790s, the time of the formation of a significant evangelical party within the Church of England and of the rise to civic prominence of many members of Nonconformist denominations with an evangelical outlook, such as Quakers and Unitarians. Reacting against the empty doctrine and formal ritual of the Church and the idle decadence of the upper classes, evangelicals, both Anglican and Nonconformist, called for the practice of a more serious and 'vital' religion. Being acutely aware of the sinfulness of the human condition and the necessity for repentance, they set high moral standards for themselves and others, which led them to be greatly concerned with the moral character of those whom they employed as workers in their businesses and servants in their homes.[20] The sudden concern of hospital governors with the moral character of their nurses during this period can therefore be explained by the increased representation of these attitudes on the hospital boards, as evangelicalism spread particularly among the mercantile and manufacturing classes from which hospital governors mostly came.

The fate of the numerically insignificant but more historically visible hospital nurses can provide an indication of how the perception of the vastly more numerous domestic nurses was changing, for it follows that the same increased expectations among employers would have led to the same dissatisfaction with their moral standing. It is significant that an early article complaining about the quality of nurses, often cited in traditional histories as the first proposal for nurse training in Britain, appeared in the *Christian Observer*, the organ of the evangelical party of the Church of England, and it was clearly motivated by the concern of the private employer. The article took the form of a review of a tract by a French Abbé on training attendants for the sick. The author of the review quoted the Abbé to remind his readers that 'the powers of medicine without good nursing, are proverbially of little avail'; furthermore, 'the chief object to a sick man [sic]' is 'his future existence' in the next life, and 'who, in such a case but would desire to have around him persons imbued with the same principles?' And yet respectable people without a family at hand to take care of them were forced in cases of illness to surrender to the care of paid nurses who as a class were characterized by '*ivrognerie*', '*malpropreté*', '*rapacité*', and '*inhumanité*' (drunkenness, impropriety, greed, and inhumanity). Taking his cue from the Abbé, the review author suggested that every hospital should set up a nurse-training school in which 'any respectable female, who wishes to learn "the art" of nursing' could receive instruction, 'and, if found competent, should be entitled to a certificate of her ability and moral deportment'. The author's objective, then, was to enable prospective employers, such as himself (he signed the article 'Invalid'), to engage respectable and technically proficient sick attendants, and so his concern was similar to that which we inferred for the hospital governors. But the author was not just hoping for morally better women to undertake nursing: he thought that nursing itself might become something morally better. He envisaged the care of the sick not as casual manual labour, undertaken from financial necessity, but something a woman might adopt as 'her chosen profession', spending six months or a year of training towards that end.[21] In other words, his proposal depended on a new concept of nursing.

This new concept of nursing, involving vocation and training, was also fundamental to the plans of the other nursing reforms listed in the traditional histories. The precise aim was different in each case, but in general they differed from that of the writer in the *Christian Observer* in that the new nurses were intended not for the satisfaction of middle-class employers but for the charitable care of the poor and outcast. The plans were mostly for the foundation of religious sisterhoods, on the model of the Sisters of Charity or the Béguines, which were very different in their formal organization (the Sisters of Charity took lifelong vows binding them to their Order, whereas the Béguines remained lay women, frequently returning to worldly life after some years), but crucially alike in being based on the religious desire of certain middle- and upper-class women to devote themselves to the care of the sick poor, nursing them in public hospitals or in their own homes. Between 1825 and 1850, there were three main initiatives for the foundation of sisterhoods in Britain by identifiable small groups, and a series of initiatives by men and women associated with the Oxford Movement. We will now look at each of these in turn.

The first of these initiatives was made in the late 1820s by a group of three men. One was Alexander Dallas, an Anglican clergyman; in 1826 he wrote an open letter to the Bishop of London entitled 'Protestant Sisters of Charity'. Another was his friend Robert Gooch, then a rising obstetrician; he wrote an article with the same title which appeared in *Blackwood's Magazine* at the end of 1825, and a little later a letter on the same theme which appeared in the *London Medical Gazette*. The third member of this group was Robert Southey, the man of letters, who knew the others because his brother Henry had been a medical student with Gooch at Edinburgh. Southey discussed the subject at length in the course of his 1829 *Colloquies on the Progress and Prospects of Society*, and he reprinted Gooch's articles as an appendix to the book. The original plan of these three men was to obtain the patronage of the Bishop of London in setting up a charitable nursing sisterhood in the Church of England. In this they were not successful, but from their writings we can see what they would have liked to do, and why.[22]

Alexander Dallas was the son of a man of letters, and had spent the early part of his career in government office, being active at home and abroad during the Napoleonic Wars. Afterwards, now in his late twenties, he contemplated taking up a profession, and after considering the Bar for a time he eventually went to Oxford with the intention of taking Holy Orders. It is clear from this that he had no special sense of vocation to the ministry at this time; he was simply looking for a career, and had decided on the Church. While he was at Oxford, however, he turned steadily more and more evangelical.[23] As a parish priest, he took a very serious view of his duties; his diary records extreme feelings of guilt when he had failed to visit his flock as much as he thought necessary.[24] Like other evangelical clergymen, Dallas had a deep – almost compulsive – concern for the spiritual welfare of the poor, and by his frequent visits and closer contact with them he was made aware of their material needs too. In particular, he noticed the difficulty which they faced in time of sickness; it was a rural area, the parish surgeon was distant and overworked, and his assistant was a poor substitute. It was because of this experience that chance encounters with the Sister of Charity and the Béguines struck him so forcibly. Protestant England, he reasoned, thanks to the revival of religious fervour, now had missionary organizations like the Catholic countries; it was time that they should also have Sisters of Charity: orders of women, animated by religious commitment, taking it as their mission to care for the needs of the sick poor.[25]

Dallas's aim, in other words, was one of philanthropy or Christian charity, which like missionary activity was for Evangelicals a way of showing forth their active faith in the world – 'living in the light', as Quakers put it.[26] Of course philanthropy and missionary activity were not entirely distinct; performing good works among the poor provided increased opportunities for spreading the Gospel. Gooch, for example, clearly intended his Protestant Sisters of Charity to provide not just for the bodily welfare of the poor, but for their spiritual welfare too. In one of his first parishes he had started a Charitable Clothing Society, of which he wrote in his diary:

> The ostensible object, that of clothing the naked, is in fact only secondary to that of getting my flock into the habit of coming to church, that they may be fed with the spiritual food which they want inducement to desire.[27]

Even the evangelical campaigns for the abolition of slavery were motivated in part by a belief that freeing the slaves was a precondition of them achieving spiritual salvation. But it would be wrong to think of evangelicals' concern for the freedom of slaves or the material welfare of the poor as ungenuine or wholly secondary to the desire to evangelize them. They saw the relief of the poor and miserable as part of God's work and a good in itself, even if a lesser good than working directly for their spiritual salvation. Dallas wrote of his Clothing Society: 'May God bless *both* its objects!' (my emphasis), and he no doubt felt similarly about the proposed Protestant Sisters of Charity.

Robert Gooch's relationship with evangelicalism was more complex. He was the son of a Yarmouth sea captain, who had been apprenticed to a local surgeon-apothecary, taken an Edinburgh MD, and spent the early part of his career as a general practitioner in Croydon (then in open country, not a suburb of London, as it is today). By the late 1820s, with the assistance of much string-pulling by his powerful patrons, he had set himself up as a specialist in midwifery and diseases of women.[28] At this time, perhaps prompted by the death of his favourite child and his own ill-health, he was turning towards vital religion. There is no record of any evangelical conversion but his diary shows him attending and approving a sermon given by the evangelical preacher Thomas Chalmers,[29] and his plea for the foundation of a nursing sisterhood was significantly addressed to

> that class of Christians in whom, above all others, religion is not a mere Sunday ceremony, but the daily and hourly principle of their thoughts and actions, and of whom I have only to complain for a little error in doctrine and more than a little cant at least in language.[30]

If he was not a whole-hearted evangelical, then, he certainly believed in serious and committed Christianity. It was to the spirit of Christian charity that he appealed in his articles on nursing, although he also drew on his medical experience to report certain cases in which unnecessary suffering or death were attributable to the failure of nurses to follow complex or awkward instructions, and he argued that religious devotion would ensure a constantly reliable standard of nursing.[31]

Robert Southey agreed with Gooch and Dallas on the need for religious zeal and commitment, shown forth in action, and he too saw care for the sick as an important part of Christian charity. The denominational tone of his appeal, however, was different. As a youth in the 1790s, he had been something of a radical in politics and a deist or unitarian in religion, but by 1830 he had become a Tory and a defender of the established

Church.[32] Like others who formed the High Church movement at this time, he was fearful of the growing power of dissent and radicalism, and sought to bring the strongest elements of their appeal into the service of the Church of England.[33] For example, the radical programme for a system of national education was something which he supported, as long as the national education was to be in the hands of the Church of England, and not in the hands of dissenters, radicals, or atheists.[34] Again, he admired Methodism for its strong basis in popular feeling and its contact with the common people, and his *Colloquies* advocated 'methodising' the Church of England so as to regain the support of people who would otherwise leave it to become Methodists.[35] The foundation of a nursing sisterhood was for him a similar project to these: one of *both* doing good works, showing faith, *and* of religious education, bringing the gospel (as interpreted by the Church of England) closer to the people.

It should now be clear why Dallas, Gooch, and Southey should have agreed on the need for a body of agents who would provide philanthropic care and spiritual guidance for the sick poor. What is not so immediately apparent is why they thought that these agents had to be women. Retrospectively this decision seems obvious, because we think of them as promoters of nursing reform, and nurses (not counting the male orderlies in military hospitals)[36] were universally female. We must remember that there was no necessity for Dallas, Gooch, and Southey to follow in this tradition, for they envisaged their agents doing work quite different from that of a nurse of the time, or even that of the Sisters of Charity and Béguines who were their explicit models. Dallas thought of them as paramedics, stand-ins for the Poor Law surgeon; Gooch intended them to have a full practical (though not theoretical) knowledge of medicine, being trained not only in nursing but in diagnosis and prescription, and he referred to them as 'a set of religious female physicians'.[37] Why were these 'religious physicians' to be female, since it was certainly not necessitated by the nature of the work?

What made the decision natural, indeed automatic, was the particular forms of masculinity and femininity which had developed among the evangelical middle class, based on the new separation of work-place and living-place and the consequent division between a male, harsh, and competitive world of business and a female, spiritual, and nurturing world of home. Philanthropy was coming to be included within women's sphere: since its main elements were religious feeling and caring and nurturing, it was possible to see it as an extension of women's domestic role.[38] With their commitment to vital religion, whether evangelical or High Church, we can take it that Dallas, Gooch, and Southey saw the Sisters of Charity and the Béguines as model examples of women doing philanthropy of a distinctively female kind – tending the sick. It was this which they hoped to promote and bring to bear on the problem of the rural sick poor. The question of gender therefore never arose, and the religious organization which they proposed was one specifically for women.

When they failed to interest the Bishop of London or other leaders of the Church of England, Dallas, Gooch, and Southey turned to the Dissenters – a relatively easy move for Dallas and Gooch, for there was little gap between evangelical Anglicans and Dissenters at this time, with much easy collaboration in missionary and anti-slavery societies. They especially hoped to arouse the interest of two Quaker women, the first being Elizabeth Fry, who at that time was at the height of her fame for her work in prison reform, and the second Amelia Opie, who was also noted for her charitable work in prisons, hospitals, and workhouses. Southey seems to have preferred Opie, who was a very untypical Quaker; while she had given up writing novels when she joined the Society of Friends, she continued to be a socialite and to enjoy the good life, which presumably made her closer to him in spirit and hence a more suitable collaborator.[39] Together, they set up a nurse-training institution in Liverpool; it lasted only two years, however, breaking up apparently because of internal divisions, since some of those involved wanted the trained nurses to be available for the upper classes to hire.[40] Dallas and Gooch meanwhile had some correspondence with Elizabeth Fry, and she expressed interest in their proposal,[41] but she was unable to do anything at that time, being preoccupied not only with the issue of prison reform but with the practical effects of her husband's bankruptcy. It was not until 1840 therefore that she embarked on the foundation of a nursing organization in London, which she did without the assistance of Dallas and Gooch. She did, however, propose to call it by their name, 'The Protestant Sisters of Charity', though on criticism that this sounded Papist the name was changed to 'The Institute of Nursing Sisters'.[42]

Elizabeth Fry's interest in nursing was essentially similar to her interest in prison reform, both deriving from a new attitude to the poor which originated among evangelicals – Anglican and Non-Conformist – at the end of the eighteenth century. Evangelicals believed that all had sinned and deserved damnation, but they also believed that all might be saved. This had a social meaning, appropriate to a newly mobile society: the poor and outcast, no matter how mean and degraded, could be raised from their low and wretched condition by an internal change analogous to the acceptance of salvation – the reformation of character. The proper attitude to the poor and outcast therefore was not to treat them and judge them by their present situation but to enable them to rise above it. In the case of lunatics, it was the aim of Samuel Tuke and the other Quakers who founded the York Retreat that they should not be treated like the brute beasts they appeared to be, but should be restored to sanity by moral therapy.[43] In the case of the sick, evangelical hospital governors tried to reform and re-educate, and not merely care for, the inmates of their institutions by introducing strict disciplinary codes or displaying improving messages on the ward walls,[44] while John Copeley Lettsom and other founders of dispensaries (many of whom were Quakers) sought to provide a means of restoring the sick poor to productive independence without the quasi-feudal relationship with a patron-governor entailed by entering a hospital.[45] In the case of criminals, it was a fundamental principle of Elizabeth Fry's prison work that the proper purpose of prisons was not to *punish* offenders but to *reform* them.[46]

Elizabeth Fry observed that a criminal was actually impeded from reforming and becoming a decent respectable citizen by the social environment within prisons, which were characterized by all kinds of immoral behaviour, such as swearing, gambling, fighting, begging, singing and dancing, looking at pornography, and sexual abuse. She believed that middle-class women had the power to assist prisoners – female prisoners in particular – to reform themselves, and she defended the suitability of such philanthropic work for women on account of their special qualities: 'their gentleness, their natural sympathy with the afflicted, their quickness of discernment, their openness to religious impressions'.[47] Her approach was to form committees of lady visitors, who would take it on themselves first to convince the inmates of 'the danger and misery of vice, the beauty of holiness, and the innumerable advantages which attach to a life of sobriety, industry, honesty and virtue',[48] and secondly to institute and maintain a system of discipline which would discourage immoral behaviour and promote cleanliness, tidiness, and good order. Scripture readings and religious instruction were an important part of this system, yet we can see that her aim was not merely the *spiritual* salvation of the inmates, but what we might call their *social* salvation: that they might be 'rescued from a condition of depravity and wretchedness, and restored to happiness, as a useful and respectable member of the community'.[49]

Evangelical concern for the sick poor was therefore just one aspect of a more general concern for the socially outcast. When the German clergyman Theodore Fliedner, inspired by Fry's work, started a Protestant order of deaconesses at Kaiserwerth, his aim was to provide Christian care not only for the sick, but for the orphans, poor children in need of schooling, the handicapped, the mentally ill, and discharged convicts (who needed special help and encouragement to go straight).[50] The Kaiserwerth deaconesses, however, as well as running schools, orphanages, and hospitals, nursed the poor in their own homes, and when Fry started her own institute, this was a feature which she imitated. She had already considered applying the principles of her work on prisons to hospitals, workhouses, lunatic asylums – any institution where the poor and wretched were accumulated in large numbers[51] – but presumably she felt that, where institutions were dubious, it was better for outcasts to be returned to society without having to enter one at all. The nurses of her institute, although hospital-trained, were to look after the poor in their own homes.[52]

By contrast, St John's House, the other famous and successful nurse-training institution of the 1840s, was very much intended to provide nurses for hospitals, and for the hospital attached to King's College, London, in particular. There were two men principally behind its foundation, one being Robert Bentley Todd, who was the first Professor of Physiology and Anatomy at the King's College medical school; he had been one of those responsible for setting up the associated hospital, and as well as acting as one of its physicians he constantly pressed for its expansion and development. The other was his friend and colleague William Bowman, Demonstrator in Anatomy at the medical school and surgeon at the hospital, who collaborated with Todd on various projects, including the *Cyclopedia of Anatomy and Physiology*, and the *Anatomy and Physiology of Man.* They clearly intended the St John's House Sisterhood to have a close relationship with their own institution; virtually from the start, it was at the King's College Hospital that the St John's House nurses received their training, and by 1856 St John's House nurses were doing all the nursing there.[53]

King's College, London, had been founded by Tory High Churchers in opposition to the radical, secular University College, with a charter which specified that 'instruction in the doctrines and duties of Christianity as taught by the Church of England should be for ever combined with other branches of useful education'.[54] Simply from the fact that Todd and Bowman held chairs at King's College, London, during its earliest years, we can infer that they subscribed to its foundational principle that Anglican religion was a central and essential part of education. Todd in particular was concerned for the pastoral care of students, and he was largely responsible for the introduction of a tutorial system to that end. He also founded scholarships for medical students, to qualify for which they had to answer questions on the Church catechism and Butler's *Analogy of Religion.*[55] Both Todd and Bowman, when their turn came to address the medical students at the start of the academic year, quoted as a cardinal principle the section of the King's College foundation document which declared

> That every system of general education for the youth of a Christian community ought to comprise instruction in the Christian religion as an indispensable part, without which the acquisition of other branches of knowledge will be conducive neither to the happiness of the individual, nor to the welfare of the State.[56]

In other words, they saw instruction in Christianity as essential to life in a Christian community. For King's College Hospital to be a Christian community, religiously correct nurses were necessary. The regulations governing St John's House were drawn up to this end: all the trainees were required to be baptized members of the Church of England; they were placed under the day-to-day direction of a clergyman Master, whose duties specifically included their religious instruction; and they were organized in a severe hierarchy, with the lowest grades being very much on trial, and promotion depending on efficiency, respectability, and devotion.[57]

The other members of the St John's House governing committee had a very similar religious allegiance and commitment to that of Todd and Bowman.[58] The Committee was under the patronage and presidency of the Bishop of London – not the former Bishop who had been so unhelpful to Dallas, Gooch, and Southey, but Bishop Blomfield, who was already becoming famous for his encouragement of the building and endowment of new churches and schools throughout London. Also on the Committee was Frederick Dennison Maurice: once a unitarian, now an Anglican professor at King's (his complex religious position had not yet prompted his expulsion) and a Christian socialist; that is to say he believed, with socialists, that the radical reform of society was necessary, but he held that this reform should be guided by Christian principles rather than those of atheistic secularism. Then there was Samuel Roffey Maitland, a man of letters, who began life as a Congregationalist but gradually became more orthodox and eventually took Holy Orders; he was working energetically for the conversion of Jews to Christianity, and since 1835 he had been first a leading contributor and then editor of the High Church Tory *British Magazine.* John William Cunningham was unusual on the Committee in being an evangelical, but from a High Church point of view he was safely and unimpeachably Anglican; as a young clergyman he had been associated with the Clapham Sect, had been made a life governor of the Church Missionary Society, and was later to become editor of the *Christian Observer.* The Committee also included Christopher Wordsworth – not the famous Master of Trinity College, Cambridge, but his son of the same name, who was Headmaster of Harrow, and noted for his work there in establishing discipline, building a school chapel, and generally injecting a religious tone into the life of the school. The other members included two colleagues of Todd and Bowman from the King's College medical school. All of those on whom information is readily available were strongly committed to the defence of the Church of England, and were noted elsewhere for their active attempts to inject Christian principles and Christian responsibility into the lives of ordinary citizens.[59]

While St John's House was being established, other sisterhoods were being founded by High Churchers who were part of the Oxford Movement associated with Edward Pusey and John

Henry Newman. The motive for the foundations in this case is clear. Members of the Oxford Movement sought to strengthen and defend the Church of England by promoting its spiritual regeneration through such means as the revival of ancient (hence more authentically Christian) forms of worship. These were taken to include full-scale religious orders, which allowed worshippers to make the extreme self-sacrifice of devoting their entire life to the service of God, binding themselves to an Order by a vow.[60] Orders of women devoted to good works seemed least likely to arouse public antagonism, and so the first Order founded by the Oxford Movement, with the cautious support of Bishop Blomfield, was a Sisterhood of Mercy, intended as a memorial to Robert Southey; this was the Park Village West community, started near Regent's Park in 1844. A few years later, with Pusey's encouragement, Priscilla Lydia Sellon began founding communities in the Plymouth area to undertake a whole range of philanthropic activities, including a school for pauper children, an orphanage, a home for delinquent boys, and a penitentiary for the reclamation of prostitutes.[61] The range of activities indicates that for the High Church sisterhoods, as for Elizabeth Fry and the Kaiserwerth deaconnesses, nursing of the sick was part of the more general enterprise of Christian philanthropy. These Orders, however, all suffered from two difficulties specific to their High Church denomination. The first difficulty was internal, and it arose because of the strong tradition of regarding contemplation as the highest form of devotion; thus in many Orders there was a conflict between those who wanted a severe restrictive rule and a retreat from the world and those wanting to do good works.[62] The second difficulty was the hostility of most people to religious Orders on the grounds that they were Papist – a suspicion amply confirmed by the members' embarrassing tendency to convert to Roman Catholicism.

Despite such denominational differences, there were certain basic similarities between all the nursing sisterhoods, actual or projected, which we have examined. First and most obviously, they were all motivated by vital religion – evangelical Anglican, Nonconformist or High Church – with nursing of the sick being just one possible form of philanthropy, a way of serving God and making faith manifest. Second, they were directed towards the spiritual and social as well as physical salvation of the sick poor, this emphasis on reclamation being part of a more general change in attitude towards social outcasts at this time. Third, in allocating this work of salvation to women, men were seeing women as providers of spirituality and loving care and women were correspondingly believing themselves possessed of these special powers – one aspect of the form of femininity which originated in middle-class evangelicalism. The aim of mobilizing women in the philanthropic reclamation of the sick poor might have been pursued in various ways; the people we have considered were led to found sisterhoods because they focused on the role of the nurse. Like Mary Stanley, the chief speaker for nursing sisterhoods in the 1850s, they were asking themselves 'at what points light can be diffused, – in what way the poor can be reached', and had thought that, as far as the sick poor were concerned, nurses might be enlisted, for they 'have access at all times, and . . . without adding to their labour, may give words of Christian comfort as they see fit'. The problem which they faced was that most nurses were wholly unsuitable for this job on account of their 'drunkenness' and 'profligacy', and the fact that 'only a very low class of women apply for the situation'.[63] Thus these reformers were driven to create a new kind of nurse who would be suitable for this new kind of work: one who was religiously motivated and who carried the trappings, at the very least, of middle-class respectability.

The number of people involved in the foundation or operation of nursing sisterhoods was very small; the reason for devoting so much attention to them is that they were chiefly responsible for the creation of this new ideal of what a nurse should be. We must now consider how their new ideal was received by the population generally. Around 1830, to judge by the difficulty Dallas, Gooch, and Southey experienced in winning support for their project, it seems to have aroused little interest or enthusiasm. In the 1840s and 1850s, however, it was taken up, assimilated and re-transmitted throughout the middle and upper classes of society with great speed and thoroughness. As a leading mediator of middle-class ideals, Charles Dickens played an important part in this process by the creation in 1843 of his character Sarah Gamp, who was the nurse of the times as judged and condemned by the new standards. As the new ideal spread, so the existing nurses became the bad 'old' nurses, relegated to an era that was now passing away, as in this feature from the *Medical Times and Gazette* in 1852:

> A paid nurse of the old school! We in the Profession well know what that means, – a hard-minded, ignorant, lazy, drunken woman, who upsets the whole establishment with her whims; sleeps when she should be awake; is cross when she should be patient; and is constant only in a persevering attempt to make the job as lucrative as possible.

The ideal was so thoroughly assimilated that it was forgotten that there had been any change, which made the general absence of attempts at nursing reform seem strange. 'Society may perhaps feel both astonished and alarmed when we assert, that within a few years only has any attempt, however slight, been made to establish institutions for the education of this important class.' The author referred in particular to the Institute of Nursing Sisters and St John's House, which were the two institutions at this date considered to be turning out 'proper' nurses of the new type.[64]

Why did the new ideal of the nurse spread so easily and rapidly? The answer surely lies in the fact that it overlapped with another ideal, that of domestic femininity, which was itself partly the product of evangelicalism and by this time had become firmly established as an essential part of middle-class respectability. The concept of woman as spiritual, caring, and possibly involved in worthy philanthropy outside the home, which as we have seen was crucial in the tacit decision of sisterhood founders that it should be women ministering to the sick poor, was now widespread and allowed easy circulation of the new sisterhood-based ideal of the nurse. But we must note that it was *only* those aspects which overlapped with the ideal of middle-class femininity which achieved general currency. The skill and knowledge of the new nurses, an important part of some at least of the sisterhood proposals, was not much stressed; as for them being trained for diagnosis and prescription, as Gooch had wanted, that was out of the question. Even the toughness and assertiveness which a nursing sister would often need when educating or disciplining rough working-class people was forgotten. What remained of the new ideal was its gentle, sympathetic, loving, and caring aspect. The ideal nurse, in short, was made over in the image of the ideal middle-class wife and mother, and indeed the two ideals were sometimes identified. Mrs Beeton, in her best-selling domestic guide for the upwardly socially mobile, declared that 'the main requirements [of a sick-nurse] are good temper, compassion for suffering, sympathy with sufferers, *which most women worthy of the name possess*, neat-handedness, quiet manners, love of order, and cleanliness' (my emphasis).[65]

The career of Florence Nightingale perfectly illustrates the power of the feminine ideal in forming the new ideal of the nurse. Her fame depended on the fact that nursing itself had become a major political issue in the 1850s, as a result of William Howard Russell's exposé of the poor standard of care which wounded British soldiers were receiving at the military hospital at Scutari. It was his unflattering comparison to the standard of care received by the French soldiers which gave rise to the famous letter in *The Times* asking 'why have we no Sisters of Charity?' and to the Secretary at War's request that Florence Nightingale should take a party of nurses to Scutari.[66] The Nightingale legend grew up during the two years that she spent in the East; the public at home, desperate for something to celebrate, eagerly believed and transmitted it, and the War Office, anxious to divert attention from the disastrous conduct of the war, orchestrated it by starting a Nightingale Fund to set up a training institution for nurses. The legend portrayed her as the Lady with the Lamp: an angelic figure, dedicated to the care of the sick, compassionate, tender, gentle, sympathetic, and selfless (specifically, refusing payment for her work); in other words, the very incarnation of middle-class domestic femininity.[67] The power of this ideal was such that a very few facts could be puffed up into a legend with a life of its own. It is significant that the many pictures of Florence Nightingale in circulation before her return were all wholly imaginary, for her family would not release her portrait; artists did not need to know what she looked like in order to represent the feminine ideal.[68]

The real Florence Nightingale was very different from the legend. Though she might be imagined as a model of domestic-minded femininity, in her unpublished 'Suggestions for Thought to Searchers after Religious Truth' she was strong in condemnation of middle-class family life for the useless idleness to which it consigned women.[69] She went to Scutari not to soothe the sufferings of wounded soldiers but to run a system of patient care and to reform the administration of the hospital. Far from being meek and selfless, in all her doings she was insistent on having control and on her power and authority being respected.[70] She had little interest in the Fund which had been started in her name or in setting up a nurse-training school; her true interest was in hygiene and public health, and nurses had significance for her only in so far as they might act as agents of sanitation.[71] She had little to do with the Nightingale school after its foundation, for she was more concerned with matters of hospital design (on which she became the leading British authority) and the reform of the army medical service.

Florence Nightingale, in short, was not a nurse. The legend about her is essentially untrue, and we would do well to remember that the Florence Nightingale of folk history is just as much a fictional character as Sarah Gamp. Yet the legend was and continues to be powerful – as powerful as the middle-class ideal of femininity from which it came. It was extremely useful to those matrons and sisters who fought for their professional status;[72] today, nurses find it a severe liability, reinforcing all too well an image of nursing which has brought them low pay and subordination to the traditionally male medical profession. For, despite being untrue, the legend is bound up with a real historical event: a change in the concept of the nurse from a lower-class domestic servant to a respectable, dedicated medical auxiliary: the ideological origin, in middle-class religion, respectability, and gender ideals, of the modern nurse.

Notes

1. At the time of writing, the reverse side of the British £10 note shows Florence Nightingale on the wards at Scutari, with her lamp – no merely practical device for seeing in the dark – radiating light across the entire picture. For an example of the children's books which transmit the story to the next generation, see L. Du Garde Peach, *Florence Nightingale* (Loughborough, 1959), still in print with Ladybird Books.

2. M. Adelaide Nutting and Lavinia L. Dock, *A History of Nursing*, 4 vols (New York, 1907); Lucy Ridgely Seymer, *A General History of Nursing* (London, 1932); Brian Abel-Smith, *A History of the Nursing Profession* (London, 1960); Vern L. Bullough and Bonnie Bullough, *The Care of the Sick: The Emergence of Modern Nursing* (London, 1979); Josephine A. Dolan, M. Louise Fitzpatrick, and Eleanor Krohn Hermann, *Nursing in Society: A Historical Perspective* (Philadelphia, 1983).

3. This was the view put forward by Celia Davies in the introduction to her *Rewriting Nursing History* (London, 1980), pp. 11–17.

4. See, for example, Davies, ibid.; Christopher Maggs, *The Origins*

of General Nursing (London, 1983); Christopher Maggs (ed.), *Nursing History: The State of the Art* (London, 1987); Rosemary White, *The Effects of the National Health Service on the Nursing Profession 1948–1961* (London, 1985); Anne Summers, *Angels and Citizens: British Women as Military Nurses 1854–1914* (London, 1988).

5. M. S. Newby, 'Florence Nightingale a woman of all-time: myths and stereotypes', *Society for the Social History of Medicine Bulletin*, 18 (1976), 5–8; Elvi Whittaker and Virginia Olesen, 'The faces of Florence Nightingale: functions of the heroine legend in an occupational sub-culture', in Robert Dingwall and Jean McIntosh (eds), *Reading in the Sociology of Nursing* (Edinburgh, London, and New York, 1978), pp. 19–35; F. B. Smith, *Florence Nightingale: Reputation and Power* (London, 1982); Monica E. Baly, *Florence Nightingale and the Nursing Legacy* (London, 1986).

6. When I wrote this chapter, an account of this kind simply did not exist. Now happily we have *An Introduction to the Social History of Nursing* by Robert Dingwall, Anne Marie Rafferty, and Charles Webster (London, 1988); also Judith Moore, *A Zeal For Responsibility: The Struggle for Professional Nursing in Victorian England, 1868–1883* (Athens, Georgia, 1988), which provides three case studies of professional conflict between nurses and doctors.

7. Herbert Butterfield, *The Whig Interpretation of History* (London, 1931). The issues raised by Butterfield are taken much further in a pair of important historiographical articles by Adrian Wilson and Timothy Ashplant: 'Whig history and present-centred history' and 'Present-centred history and the problem of historical knowledge', *The Historical Journal*, 31 (1988), 1–16, 253–74.

8. Davies, *Rewriting Nursing History*, p. 11.

9. The census report for England and Wales for 1861 lists under female occupations 2797 nurses in hospitals and lunatic asylums, 67,785 nurses described as 'domestic servant', and 24,821 nurses described as 'not domestic servant' though they are still classified with them.

10. The title was retained from the pre-Reformation hospitals which had been run by religious orders.

11. Courtney Dainton, *The Story of England's Hospitals* (London, 1961), p. 70; A. Delbert Evans and L. G. Redmond Howard, *The Romance of the British Voluntary Hospital Movement* (London, n.d.), p. 225; Guenter B. Risse, *Hospital Life in Enlightenment Scotland: Care and Teaching at the Royal Infirmary of Edinburgh* (Cambridge, 1986), pp. 41, 76; H. C. Cameron, *Mr Guy's Hospital 1726–1948* (London, 1954), p. 62.

12. William Brockbank, *Portrait of a Hospital 1752–1848: To Commemorate the Bi-Centenary of the Royal Infirmary, Manchester* (London, 1952), p. 33.

13. Dainton, *The Story of England's Hospitals*, p. 105.

14. Brockbank, *Portrait of a Hospital*, pp. 85–6.

15. Dainton, *The Story of England's Hospitals*, pp. 105–6.

16. E. M. McInnes, *St Thomas's Hospital* (London, 1963), p. 115.

17. Ibid., p. 116.

18. Cameron, *Mr Guy's Hospital*, pp. 193–4.

19. I. Bradley, *The Call to Seriousness: The Evangelical Impact on the Victorians* (London, 1976); F. K. Brown, *Fathers of the Victorians: the Age of Wilberforce* (Cambridge, 1961).

20. Pamela Horn, *The Rise and Fall of the Victorian Servant* (Gloucester, 1986), ch. 3; J. Jean Hecht, *The Domestic Servant Class in Eighteenth-Century England* (London, 1956), ch. 3.

21. *Christian Observer*, 19 (1820), 519–20.

22. [Alexander Dallas], 'Protestant Sisters of Charity: A Letter Addressed to the Lord Bishop of London, Developing a Plan for Improving the Arrangements at Present Existing for Administering Medical Advice, and Visiting the Sick Poor' (London, 1826); [Robert Gooch], 'Protestant Sisters of Charity', *Blackwood's Magazine*, 18 (1825), 732–5; 'Medical attendance on the country poor', *London Medical Gazette*, 1 (1827–8), 55–8, 151–4; Robert Southey, *Sir Thomas More: or Colloquies on the Progress and Prospects of Society*, 2nd edn, 2 vols (London, 1831; 1st edn, 1829), vol. 2, pp. 226–42, 337–56.

23. *Dictionary of National Biography*, s.v. 'Alexander R. C. Dallas'; *Incidents in the Life and Ministry of the Rev. Alex R. C. Dallas*, by his widow (London, 1871), pp. 176–88.

24. *Life of Dallas*, p. 199: see also pp. 224–5.

25. Dallas, letter; also Gooch, 'Protestant Sisters of Charity', p. 732.

26. Kathleen Heasman, *Evangelicals in Action: An Appraisal of Their Social Work in the Victorian Era* (London, 1962); Brian Harrison, 'Philanthropy and the Victorians', *Victorian Studies*, 9 (1965–6), 353–74; Robert Kilpatrick, '"Living in the Light": dispensaries, philanthropy and fevers in late eighteenth century London', in Andrew Cunningham and Roger French (eds), *The Medical Englightenment of the Eighteenth Century* (Cambridge, 1990); Bradley, *The Call to Seriousness*, ch. 6; Brown, *Fathers of the Victorians*, ch. 9.

27. *Life of Dallas*, p. 198.

28. W. Macmichael, *Lives of British Physicians* (London, 1830), pp. 305–24.

29. Ibid., pp. 328–30.

30. Gooch, 'Protestant Sisters of Charity', p. 734.

31. Ibid., pp. 733–4.

32. *D.N.B.*, s.v. 'Robert Southey'; Charles T. Browne, *The Life of Southey* (London, 1854); John Dennis (ed.), *Robert Southey: The Story of His Life Written in his Letters* (2nd edn, London, 1894).

33. Owen Chadwick, *The Victorian Church*, 2 vols (London, 1966, 1970), vol. 1, pp. 60–79.

34. Dennis (ed.), *Robert Southey*, pp. 353–4.

35. Browne, *Life of Southey*, pp. 255–6; Southey, *Colloquies*, vol. 1, pp. 382–9.

36. Anne Summers, 'Pride and prejudice: ladies and nurses in the Crimean War', *History Workshop Journal*, 16 (1983), 34.

37. Gooch, 'Protestant Sisters of Charity', p. 734; Gooch, 'Medical attendance on the country poor', pp. 353–4.

38. Catherine Hall, 'The early formation of Victorian domestic ideology', in Sandra Burman (ed.), *Fit Work for Women* (London, 1979),

pp. 15–32; Leonore Davidoff and Catherine Hall, *Family Fortunes: Men and Women of the English Middle Class 1780–1850* (London, 1987); F.K. Prochaska, *Women and Philanthropy in Nineteenth Century England* (Oxford, 1980); Anne Summers, 'A home from home – women's philanthropic work in the nineteenth century', in Burman, *Fit Work for Women*, pp. 33–63.

39. *D.N.B.*, s.v. 'Amelia Opie'. See Southey, *Colloquies*, vol. 2, pp. 230–1.

40. Browne, *Life of Southey*, pp. 256–7.

41. *Life of Dallas*, p. 224.

42. Nutting and Dock, *A History of Nursing*, vol. 2, p. 73; June Rose, *Elizabeth Fry: A Biography* (London: Macmillan, 1980).

43. Anne Digby, *Madness, Morality and Medicine: A Study of the York Retreat, 1796–1914* (Cambridge, 1985). See also Michel Foucault, *Madness and Civilisation: A History of Insanity in the Age of Reason* (London, 1967), ch. 9; Andrew T. Scull, *Museums of Madness: The Social Organisation of Insanity in Nineteenth-Century England* (London, 1979), chs. 1–2.

44. Cameron, *Mr Guy's Hospital*, pp. 73–8; Benjamin Golding, *An Historical Account of St Thomas's Hospital, Southwark* (London, 1819), p. 138.

45. Kilpatrick, '"Living in the Light"'.

46. Elizabeth Fry, *Observations on the Visiting, Superintending, and Government of Female Prisoners* (2nd edn, London, 1827), pp. 20–1.

47. Ibid., p. 3.

48. Ibid., pp. 16–17.

49. Ibid., p. 4.

50. Nutting and Dock, *A History of Nursing*, vol. 2, ch. 1; Seymer, *A General History of Nursing*, pp. 52–64.

51. Fry, *Observations on . . . Female Prisoners*, pp. 4–5.

52. Nutting and Dock, *A History of Nursing*, vol. 2, p. 73; Seymer, *A General History of Nursing*, pp. 65–6; Katherine Williams, 'From Sarah Gamp to Florence Nightingale: a critical study of hospital nursing systems from 1840 to 1897', in Celia Davies (ed.), *Rewriting Nursing History*, pp. 43–4, 46–7.

53. *D.N.B.*, s.v. 'Todd, Robert Bentley', Bowman, Sir William'; Nutting and Dock, *A History of Nursing*, vol. 2, pp. 79–86; Seymer, *A General History of Nursing*, pp. 69–70; Williams, 'From Sarah Gamp to Florence Nightingale', pp. 51–2, 65–9. But see also R[obert] Few, 'A history of St. John's House: with a full account of the circumstances which led to the withdrawal therefrom of the entire sisterhood: and a refutation of the charges made against the Sisters in the "Statement" issued by the Council on the 12th November and reiterated in the Letter of Mr. George William Bell (Honorary Secretary) dated the 31st December last' (3rd edn, London, 1884). Few claims that St John's House originated in a conversation between him and Todd in April 1848. This claim was made, however, in order to show that King's College Hospital had not been responsible for the foundation of St John's; this was part of an argument that the hospital council had no authority over the Sisterhood. Few was a governor of Charing Cross

Hospital, and he was clearly much involved in the foundation of St John's, but it seems that Todd's plans were already advanced by the time he spoke to him; Nutting and Dock refer to a circular letter from Todd the previous year (p. 79).

54. Charter of King's College, quoted in *University of London: The Historical Record* (London, 1912), p. 10.

55. *D.N.B.*, s.v. 'Todd, Robert Bentley', p. 913; R. B. Todd, *On the Resources of King's College London for Medical Education* (London, 1853), pp. 19–21.

56. William Bowman, *Thoughts for the Medical Student: An Introductory Address Delivered at King's College, London, October 1, 1851, On Occasion of the Opening of the Twentieth Session of the Medical Department* (London, 1851), p. 3. Todd, *On the Resources of King's College London*, p. 19.

57. Abel-Smith, *A History of the Nursing Profession*, p. 19; Williams, 'From Sarah Gamp to Florence Nightingale', p. 66.

58. The foundation programme, including a list of the members of the Committee, is reproduced in [Mary Stanley], *Hospitals and Sisterhoods* (London, 1854), p. 43.

59. *D.N.B.*, s.v. 'Blomfield, Charles James', 'Maurice, Frederick Dennison', 'Maitland, Samuel Roffey', 'Cunningham, John William, 'Wordsworth, Christopher (1807–1885)', 'Bowman, John Eddowes', 'Partridge, Richard'.

60. Chadwick, *The Victorian Church*, vol. 1, pp. 505–11.

61. Peter F. Anson and Allan Walter Campbell, *The Call of the Cloister* (London, 1964); Martha Vicinus, *Independent Women: Work and Community for Single Women 1850–1920* (London, 1985), pp. 69–73.

62. Vicinus, ibid., ch. 2; Margaret Goodman, *Experiences of an English Sister of Mercy* (London, 1862); Margaret Goodman, *Sisterhoods in the Church of England* (London, 1863).

63. [Stanley], *Hospitals and Sisterhoods*, p. 8.

64. *Medical Times and Gazette*, 4 (1852) 40–1.

65. Mrs Isabella Beeton, *Mrs Beeton's Book of Household Management* (London, 1982, facsimile of 1861 edition), p. 1017.

66. Cecil Woodham-Smith, *Florence Nightingale 1820–1910* (London, 1950), ch. 7. The letter appeared in *The Times* for 14 October 1854.

67. A point made by Newby, 'Florence Nightingale a woman of all-time'. For examples of ballad and picture, see Janet Horowitz Murray, *Strong Minded Women: And Other Lost Voices from 19th-Century England* (Harmondsworth, 1984), pp. 300–2; also Woodham-Smith, *Florence Nightingale*, pp. 234–5.

68. Woodham-Smith, *Florence Nightingale*, p. 235.

69. She wrote it in 1852 and revised it in 1859, after her return from the Crimea. An extract, 'Cassandra', is reprinted as an appendix to Ray Strachey, *The Cause: A Short History of the Women's Movement in Great Britain* (Virago edn., London, 1978; original edn, 1928).

70. This side of Nightingale is well represented in F.B. Smith's somewhat misogynist *Florence Nightingale: Reputation and Power* (London: Croom Helm, 1982).

71. Baly, *Florence Nightingale and the Nursing Legacy*, pp. 22–3. See also Charles E. Rosenberg, 'Florence Nightingale on contagion: the hospital as moral universe', in his (ed.) *Healing and History: Essays for George Rosen* (New York, 1979), pp. 116–36.

72. The pictures of nurses 'THEN' and 'NOW' (Sarah Gamp and Florence Nightingale?) which are reproduced as a frontispiece to Davies, *Rewriting Nursing History*, were taken from an 1888 issue of the *Nursing Record*, the organ of the British Nurses' Association. On the issue of professional status, see Abel-Smith, *A History of the Nursing Profession*, and Moore, *A Zeal for Responsibility*.

Index